'Hilarious and heartbreaking . . . I howled, yelped and occasionally choked with laughter . . . This book may hurt, but in an important and necessary way'   *The Times*

'Blisteringly funny, politically enraging and often heartbreaking . . . This should be a wake-up call to all who value the NHS'   *Sunday Express*

'If you are at all squeamish, I recommend you read *This is Going to Hurt* lying flat on your back. More than once on my commute, as I raced through Adam Kay's hilarious, heartbreaking book, I felt the legs begin to wobble . . . some entries are so funny, they make you howl . . . But for all the laughs in *This is Going to Hurt*, the book is also a devastating account of our National Health Service'   *Daily Telegraph*

'The humour is unflinching in its darkness . . . Yet I did laugh. A lot. Kay is a skilful, muscular writer, his narrative swinging from laugh-out-loud anecdotes to tales of sheer horror. The book's title is harrowingly apt . . . In the end, this book is a call to arms. That the NHS lost Kay is a tragedy. That this diary was written well before the Government's battle with junior doctors is more disturbing still'   *i*

'Beg, borrow or steal a copy . . . scalpel-sharp humour and searing insight . . . funny, sad and enraging'
                    Lorraine Kelly, *The Sun*

'We know that junior doctors have it rough. But it takes Kay's account of his 97-hour-week struggle to see just how rough . . . hilariously gruesome'   *Sunday Times*

'A heartening, laugh-out-loud confessional . . . At a time of anxiety over the future of the NHS, Kay's warts-and-all account will not only bring plenty of laughs but also delivers a moving report from the NHS's embattled frontline'
Financial Times

'Hilarious . . . not just laugh-out-loud funny, but precise, upsetting and utterly sobering for anyone at all connected with the NHS' **Jenny Colgan, *Spectator* Books of the Year**

'Shocking, sad, funny and alarming . . . A truly laudable book, hilarious, moving and caustic . . . The patient stories impact and linger in the mind, but so too does the question of how junior doctors have managed to put up with working as they do for so long . . . Kay's book is vital and timely' *Scotsman*

'If you read one book this year, make it Adam Kay's hilarious, horrifying, heartbreaking insight into the life of a junior doctor . . . an eye-opening and brutally funny insight into the appalling pressure upon the NHS. What a terrible loss Adam Kay is to the medical profession. But what a tremendous gain for your bookshelf' ***Daily Express***

'Adam Kay writes with scalpel-sharp wit . . . a genital-warts-and-all account of what life is really like for junior doctors . . . Witty, wise and frequently moving' *Mail on Sunday*

'I found myself laughing in horror over and over, but Kay's poignant final act brought me to tears. This is a valuable window into the life of a junior doctor that should be required reading for all' *Stylist*

'Brutally funny . . . jaw-dropping' *New Statesman*

'Hilarious and heartbreaking, shocking and satirical, Adam Kay's memoir of his career as a junior doctor is truly eye-opening and unputdownable . . . This must-read will leave you with a greater understanding of what junior doctors go through and how much we all take them, and the NHS, for granted'   *Psychologies*

'Painfully funny. The pain and the funniness somehow add up to something entirely good, entirely noble and entirely love-able'   **Stephen Fry**

'Finally, a true picture of the harrowing, hilarious and ultim-ately chaotic life of the junior doctor . . . This is a very, very funny book anchored by the day to day grind and catastrophe which constitutes the life of a medic in the modern NHS . . . I have been waiting for ages for a book about the NHS that dispenses with the normal twee whimsy and delves right down into the rich comic and tragic caves beneath, which are all too often considered too dark for human consumption – and here it is . . . blisteringly funny'   **Jo Brand**

'A funny, excoriatingly revealing, beautiful book' **Dawn French**

'*This is Going to Hurt* is moving, relevant, disturbing and – far more important than any of these previous adjectives – very, very funny'   **David Baddiel**

'A brilliant book'   **Russell Howard**

'Much like the NHS itself, this book is filled with hope, des-pair, miracles, catastrophe and acres of the sharpest gallows humour. A very funny book with a very sobering message'
                                                                  Chris Addison

'It's a rare book that makes me both cry and laugh. *This is Going to Hurt* is that book'   **Ian Rankin**

'Bloody funny'   **Minnie Driver**

'By turns witty, gruesome, alarming, and touching. Always illuminating and searingly honest'   **Jonathan Dimbleby**

'Brilliant'   **Mark Haddon**

'At once hilarious and shocking, moving and irreverent, *This is Going to Hurt* is a book that demands to be read. Adam Kay's deft comic tone is a brilliant counterpoint to his most serious of intents: to impress upon us the importance of the NHS in our lives and the irreversible damage being inflicted upon it by indifferent governments'   **Maggie O'Farrell**

'Horrifyingly hilarious and hilariously horrifying'
                                    Danny Wallace

'Unputdownable. You must read this book if you like reading, like laughing or love our NHS. It's a spit-your-tea-out-laughing clarion call to stand up for our junior doctors with all our might'   **Shappi Khorsandi**

'Absolutely adored it. Brilliant'   **Jack Whitehall**

'Kay is a brilliantly talented writer . . . Piles of this book should be in every GP surgery waiting room and A&E department in the country. Heartbreaking, dazzling, brutally honest'
                                    Bridget Christie

'This is a ferociously funny book, but beneath the sheen of brilliant one-liners is a passionate, acutely personal examination of what the health service does for us, and what we're in danger of doing to it'   **Mark Watson**

'By turns hilarious, shocking, heartbreaking and humbling'
John Niven

'Superb' **Pam Ayres**

'A scurrilously funny, poignant and fascinatingly horrific tale of being torn to pieces and spat out by the strangely loveable but graceless monster that is the NHS' **Milton Jones**

'As a hypochondriac I was worried about reading Adam Kay's book. Luckily it's incredibly funny – so funny, in fact, that it gave me a hernia from laughing' **Joe Lycett**

'What a hilarious, stomach-churning, thought-provoking heartbreaker of a book. I loved every single page'
Jill Mansell

'What an amazing book. I laughed so hard and often I nearly choked, but it's also very moving and important. Everyone should read it' **Cathy Rentzenbrink**

'This made me laugh out loud and cry in equal measures. Adam's book weaves in and out of his patients' lives and in so doing he tells, in a better narrative than I have ever seen before, of the pain and joy of working so close to despair, disease and death' **Prof. Clare Gerada MBE, past chair of the Royal College of General Practitioners**

This is Going to Hurt

Adam Kay

This is Going to Hurt

Secret Diaries of a Junior Doctor

PICADOR

First published 2017 by Picador

This paperback edition with extra material
first published 2018 by Picador
an imprint of Pan Macmillan
20 New Wharf Road, London N1 9RR
Associated companies throughout the world
www.panmacmillan.com

ISBN 978-1-5098-5863-7

Copyright © Adam Kay 2017, 2018

The right of Adam Kay to be identified as the
author of this work has been asserted by him in accordance
with the Copyright, Designs and Patents Act 1988.

All rights reserved. No part of this publication may be reproduced,
stored in a retrieval system, or transmitted, in any form, or by any means
(electronic, mechanical, photocopying, recording or otherwise)
without the prior written permission of the publisher.

Pan Macmillan does not have any control over, or any responsibility for,
any author or third-party websites referred to in or on this book.

27

A CIP catalogue record for this book is available from the British Library.

Printed and bound by CPI Group (UK) Ltd, Croydon, CR0 4YY

This book is sold subject to the condition that it shall not, by way of
trade or otherwise, be lent, hired out, or otherwise circulated without
the publisher's prior consent in any form of binding or cover other than
that in which it is published and without a similar condition including
this condition being imposed on the subsequent purchaser.

Visit **www.picador.com** to read more about all our books
and to buy them. You will also find features, author interviews and
news of any author events, and you can sign up for e-newsletters
so that you're always first to hear about our new releases.

To James

for his wavering support

And to me

without whom this book would

not have been possible

To respect the privacy of those friends and colleagues who might not wish to be recognized, I have altered various personal details. To maintain patient confidentiality, I have changed clinical information that might identify any individuals, altered dates[*] and anonymized names.[†] Although fuck knows why – they can't threaten to strike me off any more.

---

[*] I worked a lot on labour wards, and people tend to remember the dates their kids were born.

[†] I have generally used the names of minor *Harry Potter* characters, to substitute one legal nightmare for another.

Contents

Introduction   *xvii*

1. House Officer   *1*

2. Senior House Officer – Post One   *30*

3. Senior House Officer – Post Two   *61*

4. Senior House Officer – Post Three   *86*

5. Registrar – Post One   *108*

6. Registrar – Post Two   *136*

7. Registrar – Post Three   *163*

8. Registrar – Post Four   *196*

9. Senior Registrar   *231*

10. Aftermath   *257*

*An Open Letter to the
Secretary of State for Health*   *265*

Afterword   *267*

Extra Diary Entries   *271*

Acknowledgements   *279*

Introduction

In 2010, after six years of training and a further six years on the wards, I resigned from my job as a junior doctor. My parents still haven't forgiven me.

Last year, the General Medical Council wrote to me to say they were taking my name off the medical register. It wasn't exactly a huge shock, as I hadn't practised medicine in half a decade,* but I found it a big deal on an emotional level to permanently close this chapter of my life.

It was, however, excellent news for my spare room, as I cleared out box after box of old paperwork, shredding files faster than Jimmy Carr's accountant. One thing I

---

* A study by the Department of Health in 2006 found that the public (quite reasonably) believed doctors were subject to annual appraisals. The truth was, at the time, doctors could quite happily go from the day they qualified until the day they retired without anyone checking they could still remember which end of the syringe goes into the patient. Following an inquiry into the Harold Shipman case, a process of revalidation was introduced in 2012, whereby doctors are now assessed every five years. You'd be nervous about a lot of vehicles on the road if they only got an MOT every five years, but still, better than nothing I guess.

did rescue from the jaws of death was my training port-folio. All doctors are recommended to log their clinical experiences, in what's known as 'reflective practice'. On looking through this portfolio for the first time in years, my reflective practice seemed to involve going up to my hospital on-call room and writing down anything remotely interesting that had happened that day, like a medical Anne Frank (only with worse accommodation).

Among the funny and the mundane, the countless objects in orifices and the petty bureaucracies, I was reminded of the brutal hours and the colossal impact being a junior doctor had on my life. Reading back, it felt extreme and unreasonable in terms of what was expected of me, but at the time I'd just accepted it as part of the job. There were points where I wouldn't have flinched if an entry read 'swam to Iceland for antenatal clinic' or 'had to eat a helicopter today'.

Around the same time that I was reliving all this through my diaries, junior doctors in the here and now were coming under fire from politicians. I couldn't help but feel doctors were struggling to get their side of the story across (probably because they were at work the whole time) and it struck me that the public weren't hearing the truth about what it actually means to be a doctor. Rather than shrugging my shoulders and shred-ding the evidence, I decided I had to do something to redress the balance.

So here they are: the diaries I kept during my time in the NHS, verrucas and all. What it's like working on the front line, the repercussions in my personal life, and how, one terrible day, it all became too much for me. (Sorry for the spoiler, but you watched *Titanic* knowing how that was going to play out.)

Along the way, I'll help you out with the medical terminology and provide a bit of context about what each job involved. Unlike being a junior doctor, I won't just drop you in the deep end and expect you to know exactly what you're doing.

1

House Officer

The decision to work in medicine is basically a version of the email you get in early October asking you to choose your menu options for the work Christmas party. No doubt you'll choose the chicken, to be on the safe side, and it's more than likely everything will be all right. But what if someone shares a ghastly factory farming video on Facebook the day before and you inadvertently witness a mass debeaking? What if Morrissey dies in November and, out of respect for him, you turn your back on a lifestyle thus far devoted almost exclusively to consuming meat? What if you develop a life-threatening allergy to escalopes? Ultimately, no one knows what they'll fancy for dinner in sixty dinners' time.

Every doctor makes their career choice aged sixteen, two years before they're legally allowed to text a photo of their own genitals. When you sit down and pick your A levels, you're set off on a trajectory that continues until you either retire or die and, unlike your work Christmas party, Janet from procurement won't swap your chicken for her halloumi skewers – you're stuck with it.

At sixteen, your reasons for wanting to pursue a

career in medicine are generally along the lines of 'My mum/dad's a doctor', 'I quite like *Holby City*' or 'I want to cure cancer'. Reasons one and two are ludicrous, and reason three would be perfectly fine – if a little earnest – were it not for the fact that's what research scientists do, not doctors. Besides, holding anyone to their word at that age seems a bit unfair, on a par with declaring the 'I want to be an astronaut' painting you did aged five a legally binding document.

Personally, I don't remember medicine ever being an active career decision, more just the default setting for my life – the marimba ringtone, the stock photo of a mountain range as your computer background. I grew up in a Jewish family (although they were mostly in it for the food); went to the kind of school that's essentially a sausage factory designed to churn out medics, lawyers and cabinet members; and my dad was a doctor. It was written on the walls.

Because medical schools are oversubscribed ten-fold, all candidates must be interviewed, with only those who perform best under a grilling being awarded a place. It's assumed all applicants are on course for straight As at A level, so universities base their decisions on non-academic criteria. This, of course, makes sense: a doctor must be psychologically fit for the job – able to make decisions under a terrifying amount of pressure, able to break bad news to anguished relatives, able to deal with death on a daily basis. They must have something that cannot be memorized and graded: a great doctor must have a huge heart and a distended aorta through which pumps a vast lake of compassion and human kindness.

At least, that's what you'd think. In reality, medical schools don't give the shiniest shit about any of that. They don't even check you're OK with the sight of blood. Instead, they fixate on extracurricular activities. Their ideal student is captain of two sports teams, the county swimming champion, leader of the youth orchestra and editor of the school newspaper. It's basically a Miss Congeniality contest without the sash. Look at the Wikipedia entry for any famous doctor, and you'll see: 'He proved himself an accomplished rugby player in youth leagues. He excelled as a distance runner and in his final year at school was vice-captain of the athletics team.' This particular description is of a certain Dr H. Shipman, so perhaps it's not a rock-solid system.

Imperial College in London were satisfied that my distinctions in grade eight piano and saxophone, alongside some half-arsed theatre reviews for the school magazine, qualified me perfectly for life on the wards, and so in 1998 I packed my bags and embarked upon the treacherous six-mile journey from Dulwich to South Kensington.

As you might imagine, learning every single aspect of the human body's anatomy and physiology, plus each possible way it can malfunction, is a fairly gargantuan undertaking. But the buzz of knowing I was going to become a doctor one day – such a big deal you get to literally change your name, like a superhero or an international criminal – propelled me towards my goal through those six long years.

Then there I was, a junior doctor.* I could have gone on *Mastermind* with the specialist subject 'the human body'. Everyone at home would be yelling at their TVs that the subject I'd chosen was too vast and wide-ranging, that I should have gone for something like 'atherosclerosis' or 'bunions', but they'd have been wrong. I'd have nailed it.

It was finally time to step out onto the ward armed with all this exhaustive knowledge and turn theory into practice. My spring couldn't have been coiled any tighter. So it came as quite the blow to discover that I'd spent a quarter of my life at medical school and it hadn't remotely prepared me for the Jekyll and Hyde existence of a house officer.†

During the day, the job was manageable, if mind-numbing and insanely time-consuming. You turn up every morning for the 'ward round', where your whole

---

* 'Junior doctor' refers to anyone who isn't a consultant. It's a bit confusing as a lot of these 'junior doctors' are actually pretty senior – some have been working for fifteen years, picking up PhDs and various other postgraduate qualifications. It's a bit like calling everyone in Westminster apart from the prime minister a 'junior politician'.

† The hierarchy goes: house officer, senior house officer (SHO), registrar, senior registrar, consultant. They've recently renamed the ranks: it's now F1, F2, ST1–7. Everyone still uses the old terminology though, like when Coco Pops were briefly rebranded as Choco Krispies.

team of doctors pootles past each of their patients. You trail behind like a hypnotized duckling, your head cocked to one side in a caring manner, noting down every pronouncement from your seniors – book an MRI, refer to rheumatology, arrange an ECG. Then you spend the rest of your working day (plus generally a further unpaid four hours) completing these dozens, sometimes hundreds of tasks – filling in forms, making phone calls. Essentially, you're a glorified PA. Not really what I'd trained so hard for, but whatever.

The night shifts, on the other hand, made Dante look like Disney – an unrelenting nightmare that made me regret ever thinking my education was being under-utilized. At night, the house officer is given a little paging device affectionately called a bleep and responsibility for every patient in the hospital. The fucking lot of them. The night-time SHO and registrar will be down in A&E reviewing and admitting patients while you're up on the wards, sailing the ship alone. A ship that's enormous, and on fire, and that no one has really taught you how to sail. You've been trained how to examine a patient's cardiovascular system, you know the physiology of the coronary vasculature, but even when you can recognize every sign and symptom of a heart attack, it's very different to actually managing one for the first time.

You're bleeped by ward after ward, nurse after nurse with emergency after emergency – it never stops, all night long. Your senior colleagues are seeing patients in A&E with a specific problem, like pneumonia or a broken leg. Your patients are having similar emergencies, but they're hospital inpatients, meaning they already had something significantly wrong with them in the first place. It's a 'build your own burger' of symptoms layered on conditions layered on diseases: you see a patient with pneumonia who was admitted with liver failure, or a patient who's broken their leg falling out of bed after another epileptic fit. You're a one-man, mobile, essentially untrained A&E department, getting drenched in bodily fluids (not even the fun kind), reviewing an endless stream of worryingly sick patients who, twelve hours earlier, had an entire team of doctors caring for them. You suddenly long for the sixteen-hour admin sessions. (Or, ideally, some kind of compromise job, that's neither massively beyond nor beneath your abilities.)

It's sink or swim, and you have to learn how to swim because otherwise a ton of patients sink with you. I actually found it all perversely exhilarating. Sure it was hard work, sure the hours were bordering on inhumane and sure I saw things that have scarred my retinas to this day, but I was a doctor now.

Tuesday, 3 August 2004

Day one. H* has made me a packed lunch. I have a new stethoscope,† a new shirt and a new email address: atom.kay@nhs.net. It's good to know that no matter what happens today, nobody could accuse me of being the most incompetent person in the hospital. And even if I am, I can blame it on Atom.

I'm enjoying the ice-breaking potential of the story, but in the pub afterwards, my anecdote is rather trumped by my friend Amanda. Amanda's surname is Saunders-Vest. They have spelled out the hyphen in her name, making her amanda.saundershyphenvest@nhs.net.

Wednesday, 18 August 2004

Patient OM is a seventy-year-old retired heating engineer from Stoke-on-Trent. But tonight, Matthew, he's going to be an eccentric German professor with ze unconvinzing agzent. Not just tonight in fact, but this morning, this afternoon and every day of his admission;

---

* H is my short-suffering partner of six months. Don't worry – you're not going to have to remember huge numbers of characters. It's not *Game of Thrones*.

† I'm all for explaining terminology as we go along, but if you don't know what a stethoscope is, this is probably a book to regift.

thanks to his dementia, exacerbated by a urinary tract infection.*

Prof OM's favourite routine is to follow behind the ward round, his hospital gown on back-to-front, like a white coat (plus or minus underwear, for a bit of morning Bratwurst), and chip in with 'Yes!', 'Zat is correct!' and the occasional 'Genius!' whenever a doctor says something.

On consultant and registrar ward rounds, I escort him back to his bed immediately and make sure the nursing staff keep him tucked in for a couple of hours. On my solo rounds, I let him tag along for a bit. I don't particularly know what I'm doing, and I don't have vast depths of confidence even when I do, so it's actually quite helpful to have a superannuated German cheerleader behind me shouting out, 'Zat is brilliant!' every so often.

Today he took a dump on the floor next to me so I sadly had to retire him from active duty.

Monday, 30 August 2004

Whatever we lack in free time, we more than make up for in stories about patients. Today in the mess† over

---

* In the elderly, urinary tract infections, or any kind of low-grade sepsis, often make them go a bit nuts.

† The 'doctors' mess' either refers to our communal area with a few sofas and a knackered pool table or the state of most of my patients in the first few months.

lunch we're trading stories about nonsense 'symptoms' that people have presented with. Between us in the last few weeks we've seen patients with itchy teeth, sudden *improvement* in hearing and arm pain during urination. Each one gets a polite ripple of laughter, like a local dignitary's speech at a graduation ceremony. We go round the table sharing our version of campfire ghost stories until it's Seamus's turn. He tells us he saw someone in A&E this morning who thought they were only sweating from half of their face.

He sits back in anticipation of bringing the house down, but there's merely silence. Until pretty much everyone chimes in with: 'So, Horner's syndrome then?' He's never heard of it, specifically not the fact that it likely indicates a lung tumour. Seamus scrapes his chair back with an ear-splitting screech and dashes off to make a phone call to get the patient back to the department. I finish his Twix.

Friday, 10 September 2004

I notice that every patient on the ward has a pulse of 60 recorded in their observation chart so I surreptitiously inspect the healthcare assistant's measurement technique. He feels the patient's pulse, looks at his watch and meticulously counts the number of seconds per minute.

Sunday, 17 October 2004

To give myself a bit of credit, I didn't panic when the patient I was reviewing on the ward unexpectedly started hosing enormous quantities of blood out of his mouth and onto my shirt. To give myself no credit whatsoever, I didn't know what else to do. I asked the nearest nurse to get Hugo, my registrar, who was on the next ward, and meantime I put in a Venflon[*] and ran some fluids. Hugo arrived before I could do anything else, which was handy as I was completely out of ideas by that point. Start looking for the patient's stopcock? Shove loads of kitchen roll down his throat? Float some basil in it and declare it gazpacho?

Hugo diagnosed oesophageal varices,[†] which made sense as the patient was the colour of Homer Simpson – from the early series, when the contrast was much more extreme and everyone looked like a cave painting – and tried to control the bleeding with a Sengstacken

---

[*] A Venflon, or cannula, is the plastic tube that gets shoved into the back of the hand or the crook of your elbow so we can run drugs or fluids intravenously through a drip. Putting in Venflons is one of the key responsibilities of a house officer, although I got through medical school without ever having tried it. On the night before my first day as a doctor, one of my flatmates in our on-site hospital accommodation stole a box of about eighty of them from a ward and we practised cannulating ourselves for a few hours until we could finally do it. We were covered in track marks for days.

[†] Varices are a horrible complication of liver cirrhosis, where you essentially get huge varicose veins inside your oesophagus, which can rupture at any point and bleed heavily.

tube.* As the patient flailed around, resisting this awful thing going down his throat, the blood jetted everywhere: on me, on Hugo, on the walls, curtains, ceiling. It was like a particularly avant-garde episode of *Changing Rooms*. The sound was the worst part. With every breath the poor man took you could hear the blood sucking down into his lungs, choking him.

By the time the tube was inserted, he'd stopped bleeding. Bleeding always stops eventually, and this was for the saddest reason. Hugo pronounced the patient's death, wrote up the notes and asked the nurse to inform the family. I peeled off my blood-soaked clothes and we silently changed into scrubs for the rest of the shift. So there we go, the first death I've ever witnessed and every bit as horrific as it could possibly have been. Nothing romantic or beautiful about it. That sound. Hugo took me outside for a cigarette – we both desperately needed one after that. And I'd never smoked before.

Tuesday, 9 November 2004

Bleeped awake at 3 a.m. from my first half-hour's shut-eye in three shifts to prescribe a sleeping pill for a patient, whose sleep is evidently much more important than mine. My powers are greater than I realized – I arrive on the ward to find the patient is asleep.

---

* A tube you can wedge down the throat that – when it's in position – can be inflated like a balloon, to put pressure on the vessels and hopefully stop the bleeding.

Friday, 12 November 2004

An inpatient's blood results show her clotting is all over the shop for no good reason. Hugo eventually cracks it. She has been taking St John's Wort capsules from a health food shop for anxiety. Hugo points out to her (and, in fairness, me) that it interacts with the metabolism of warfarin, and her clotting will probably settle down if she stops taking it. She is astonished. 'I thought it was just herbal – how can it be that bad for you?'

At the sound of the words 'just herbal', the temperature in the room seems to drop a few degrees and Hugo barely holds in a weary sigh. It's clearly not his first time at this particular rodeo.

'Apricot stones contain cyanide,' he replies drily. 'The death cap mushroom has a fifty per cent fatality rate. Natural does not equal safe. There's a plant in my garden where if you simply sat under it for ten minutes then you'd be dead.' Job done: she bins the tablets.

I ask him about that plant over a colonoscopy later. 'Water lily.'

Monday, 6 December 2004

All junior doctors at the hospital have been asked to sign a document opting out of the European Working Time Directive* because our contracts are non-compliant with it. This week I have seen H for under two hours and worked for a grand total of ninety-seven. Non-compliant doesn't quite seem to cover it. My contract has taken the directive, dragged it screaming from its bed in the dead of night and waterboarded it.

Thursday, 20 January 2005

Dear drug-dealing scrote,

Over the last few nights, we've had to admit three young men and women – all dry as a husk, basically collapsed through hypotension, and with their electrolytes up the fuck.† The only connection between these individuals is their recent use of cocaine. For all its heart-attacking, septum-shrinking risks, cocaine does not cause

---

* The European Working Time Directive was brought in to provide some legal measure to stop employers working their staff to their bleary-eyed deaths, by limiting shifts to a 'mere' forty-eight hours per week.

† Electrolytes are the salts in the blood – mostly sodium, potassium, chloride and calcium. If levels become too high or too low, your body has a way of alerting you, by making your heart stop or putting you in a coma. It's clever like that.

this to happen to people. What I'm pretty confident is going on here – and I want a Nobel Prize or at the very least a Pride of Britain Award if I'm right – is that you've been bulking out your supply with your nan's frusemide.*

Aside from the fact you're wasting my evenings and my unit's beds, it feels like fairly terrible business practice to be hospitalizing your customers. Kindly use chalk like everyone else.

Yours faithfully, Dr Adam Kay

Monday, 31 January 2005

Saved a life tonight. I was bleeped to see a sixty-eight-year-old inpatient who was as close to death's door as it's possible to be – he'd already pressed the bell and was peering through the frosted glass into the Grim Reaper's hallway. His oxygen saturation[†] was 73 per cent – I suspect if the vending machine hadn't been out of order and I'd bought my Snickers as planned, it would have all been too late.

---

* Frusemide, or Furosemide, is a diuretic – if you've got a build-up of fluid in your lungs or tissues, generally from a malfunctioning heart or kidneys, it will make you pee it out. If you don't have a build-up of fluid, as here, it will make you pee out the water content of your blood.

† Oxygen saturation is the percentage of oxygen in your blood, and is measured by that little clip they put on the end of your finger. It should be as close to 100 per cent as possible, definitely above 90 per cent, and *definitely* definitely above 80 per cent.

14

I didn't even have the spare seconds to run through the bullet points of a management plan in my head – I just started performing action after action on an autopilot mode I didn't know I possessed. Oxygen on, intravenous access, blood tests, blood gases, diuretics, catheter. He started to perk up pretty much immediately, the bungee rope jerking him back from a millimetre above the concrete. Sorry, Death – you're one short for your dinner party this evening. By the time Hugo arrived, I felt like Superman.

A strange realization that it's the first time I've actually saved a life in five months as a doctor. Everyone on the outside imagines we roam the wards performing routine acts of heroism; I even assumed that myself when I started. The truth is, although dozens, maybe hundreds, of lives are saved every day on hospital wards, almost every time it happens it's in a much more low-key, team-based way. Not by a doctor performing a single action, so much as implementing a sensible plan which gets carried out by any number of colleagues, who at every stage check the patient is getting better and modify the plan if they're not.

But sometimes it *is* down to one person; and today, for the first time, it was me. Hugo seems happy, or at least as happy as he's capable of being: 'Well, you've bought him another couple of weeks on earth.' Come on – give a superhero a break here.

Monday, 7 February 2005

My move to surgery* has rewarded me with my very first degloving injury.†

Patient WM is eighteen and was out celebrating with friends. After chucking-out time he found himself dancing on the roof of a bus shelter, and then decided to descend to ground level using a handy neighbouring lamp post as a fireman's pole. He jumped over to the lamp post and slid down, koala-bear style. He unfortunately misjudged the texture of the lamp post – it wasn't the smooth ride he was expecting at all, but a chafing, agonizing, gritty slump to the bottom. He therefore presented to A&E with severe grazing to both palms and a complete degloving of his penis.

I have seen a lot of penises in my brief time in urology (and beyond) but this was far and away the worst one I have ever seen. Worthy of a rosette, if only there'd been a place to pin it. A couple of inches of urethra, coated with a thin layer of bloody pulp, maybe half a centimetre diameter in total. It brought to mind a remnant of spaghetti stuck to the bottom of the bowl by a

---

* House officers generally spend six months working in medicine and six months in surgery. The very shortest of straws saw me working in urology.

† A degloving injury is where skin is traumatically torn from the underlying tissues – typically seen in motorcycle accidents, where the rider's hands drag along the ground. Rats are able to deglove their tails at will to escape capture. Quite why we were taught this at medical school escapes me.

smear of tomato sauce. Perhaps not surprisingly, WM was upset. His distress was only made worse when he asked if the penis could be 'regloved'. Mr Binns, the consultant, calmly explained that the 'glove' was spread evenly up eight foot of lamp post in west London.

Monday, 21 February 2005

Discharging a patient home after laparoscopy,[*] I sign her off work for two weeks. She offers me a tenner to sign her off for a month. I laugh, but she's serious, and ups her offer to fifteen quid. I suggest she sees her GP if she's not feeling up to work after a fortnight.

I clearly need to dress smarter if that's the level of bribe I'm attracting. On the way home I wonder how much she'd have needed to offer before I said yes. Depressingly, I put it somewhere around £50.

Monday, 14 March 2005

Out for dinner with H and some mates – a pizza restaurant with exposed brickwork, too much neon, menus on clipboards, an unnecessarily complicated ordering

---

[*] Almost any abdominal operation can now be performed laparoscopically, which is Greek for 'much much slower', and involves inserting tiny cameras and instruments on long sticks through little holes. It's fiddly and takes a long time to learn. Recreate the experience for yourself by tying your shoelaces with chopsticks. With your eyes closed. In space.

system and the almost total removal of waiting staff. You're given a device that beeps and vibrates when your order is ready, whereupon you schlep across the artfully mismatched tiles to collect your pizza from a disinterested server who sits there safe in the knowledge that no one ever asks for the 12.5 per cent service charge to be taken off the bill – even when nobody actually serves you.

The device goes off, I say 'Oh my God' and reflexively jump to my feet. It's not that I'm particularly excited about my Fiorentina – it's just that the fucking thing has the exact same pitch and timbre as my hospital bleep. H takes my pulse: it's 95. Work has pretty much given me PTSD.

Sunday, 20 March 2005

There's more to breaking bad news than 'I'm afraid it's cancer' and 'We did everything we could'. Nothing can prepare you for sitting down a patient's daughter to explain that something rather upsetting happened to her frail, elderly father overnight.

I had to tell her that the patient in the bed next to her dad's became extremely agitated and confused last night. That he thought her father was in fact his own wife. That unfortunately by the time the nurses heard the commotion and attended it was too late, and this patient was straddling her father and had ejaculated onto his face.

'At least it didn't . . . go any further than that,' said the daughter, in a world-class demonstration of finding the positive in a situation.

Monday, 11 April 2005

About to take a ten-year-old straight from A&E to theatre for a ruptured appendix. Colin, a charming registrar, has been conducting a masterclass in dealing with a worried mum – explaining everything that's going on in her son's tummy, what we're going to do to fix it, how long it'll take, when he'll be allowed home. I try to absorb his method. It's about telling her just the right amount – keeping her informed but not over-whelmed – and delivering everything at the right level; not too much jargon, but never patronizing. Above all, it's about being professional and kind.

Her expression becomes less uneasy by the second and I can feel the angst leave her body like an evil spirit, or trapped wind. It's time to take the kid upstairs, so Colin nods to the mum and says, 'Quick kiss before he goes off to theatre?' She leans over and pecks Colin on the cheek. Her pride and joy is wheeled away, his own cheek sadly dry.

Tuesday, 31 May 2005

Three nights ago, I admitted patient MJ, a homeless guy in his fifties, with acute pancreatitis. This was the third time we'd admitted him with acute pancreatitis since I started this job. We got him comfortable with pain relief and started him on IV fluids – he was sore and miserable.

'At least you get a warm bed for a few nights,' I said.

'Are you joking?' he replied. 'I'll get bloody MRSA in here.' It's come to something when the streets outside a hospital have a better reputation for cleanliness than the corridors within.

I don't like to preach, but I'm a doctor and not wanting him to die is kind of in the job description, so I reminded him he's in here because of alcohol,* and even if I can't persuade him to stop drinking (I can't), could I at least ask him to stay off it until we've got him out of hospital, as that will really help. This time, it'd be a real bonus if he wouldn't mind laying off the alcogel dispensers.

He reared back like I'd just accused him of twincest, telling me that of course he would *never* do that – they've changed the recipe recently and now it tastes really bitter. He pulled me closer to whisper in my ear that in this hospital you're best off sucking on some of the sanitizing wipes, then gave me a conspiratorial tap on the arm as if to say, 'that one's on me'. Tonight he

---

* Pancreatitis is extremely painful, often very severe, and is generally caused by either alcohol or gallstones. There are a number of other causes, and the mnemonic for remembering them, pleasingly, is GET SMASHED. (The second 'S' stands for scorpion venom.)

discharged himself 'home', but will doubtless be back with us in the coming weeks.

As per tradition, I celebrate the end of our run of night shifts with my SHO, and go for a slap-up breakfast and a bottle of white wine at Vingt-Quatre. Night shifts are essentially a different time zone to the rest of the country, so even though it's 9 a.m., you can hardly call it an eye-opener – it's practically a nightcap. As I'm refilling our glasses, there's a knock on the window. It's MJ, who laughs uproariously before shooting me his best 'I knew it!' look. I resolve to sit further from the window next time. Or to just have a quick suck on an alcohol wipe in the changing rooms.

Sunday, 5 June 2005

It would be unfair to label every single orthopaedic surgeon as a bone-crunching Neanderthal simply on the basis of the 99 per cent of them it applies to, but my heart does seem to sink with every night-time bleep to their ward.

So far this weekend I've reviewed two of their patients. Yesterday: a man in atrial fibrillation* following surgery for a #NOF.† I note from his admission ECG he was in AF at that point too – a fact completely unnoticed

---

* Atrial fibrillation (AF) means the heart is beating fast, erratically and inefficiently – this isn't ideal.

† #NOF means fractured Neck of Femur. If you thought # was a hashtag, you're banned from reading the rest of the book.

by his admitting team, even though it would almost certainly explain why he ended up sprawled across the floor in Debenhams in the first place. I feel like running a teaching session for the orthopaedic department entitled, 'Sometimes people fall over for a reason'.

Today, I'm asked to review a twenty-year-old patient whose blood tests show abnormal renal function. Both his arms are in full plaster casts, like a *Scooby Doo* villain. He's got no drip for fluids and an untouched glass of water on his bedside table that – despite all the will in the world, I'm sure – physics has prevented him from touching for the past couple of days. I prescribe IV fluids for the patient, though it would be more efficient to prescribe common sense for some of my colleagues.

Tuesday, 7 June 2005

Assisting in theatres on the emergency list, removing a 'foreign object' from a patient's rectum. Less than a year as a doctor and this is the fourth object I have removed from a rectum – professionally, at least.

My first encounter was a handsome young Italian man who attended hospital with the majority of a toilet brush inside of him (bristles first), and went home with a colostomy bag. His big Italian mother was grateful in ways that Brits never are, lavishing thanks and praise on every member of staff she met for saving her son's life. She put her arm round the equally handsome young man who attended hospital with her son. 'And thank

God his friend Philip was staying in the spare room at the time to call the ambulance!'

Most of these patients suffer from Eiffel Syndrome – 'I fell, doctor! I fell!' – and the tales of how things get where can be skyscraper tall (come to think of it, it's only a matter of time before someone tries to sit on the Gherkin), but today is the first time I've actually believed the patient's story. It's a credible and painful sounding incident with a sofa and a remote control that at the very least had me furrowing my brow and thinking, 'Well, I suppose it *could* happen.' Upon removal of the remote control in theatre, however, we notice it has a condom on it, so maybe it wasn't a complete accident.

Thursday, 16 June 2005

I told a patient that his MRI wouldn't be until next week and he threatened to break both my legs. My first thought was, 'Well, it'll be a couple of weeks off work.' I was *this* close to offering to find him a baseball bat.

Saturday, 25 June 2005

Called to pronounce death* on an elderly patient – he'd been extremely sick, wasn't for resuscitation, and this wasn't unexpected. The staff nurse takes me to the

---

* Doctors are legally obliged to fill out death certificates for their patients, detailing causes of death. In hospital settings they will generally also be asked to formally pronounce (confirm) death.

cubicle, points out the slate-grey former patient and introduces me to the wife, who you could say isn't technically a widow until I make the call that he's officially dead. Nature may do all the heavy lifting, but you still need me on hand to sign the form.

I extend condolences to the patient's wife, and suggest she might want to wait outside while I perform some formalities, but she says she'd rather stay. I'm not sure why; I don't think she is either. Perhaps every moment with him matters, even if he's no longer with us, or maybe she wants to check I'm not one of those doctors she's read about in the *Mail* who does unspeakable things to the deceased. Anyway, she's settling down in her front-row seat whether I like it or not.

I've pronounced three deaths before, but this is the first time I've had a captive audience. I feel I should have laid on refreshments. She clearly doesn't realize quite how tense, silent and drawn-out this evening's performance is going to be – more Pinter than Priscilla, Queen of the Desert.

I confirm the patient's identity from his hospital wristband, check visually for respiratory effort, check there's no response to verbal or physical stimuli. Feel for a carotid pulse, check with a torch that pupils are fixed and dilated. Check watch and listen with stethoscope for heart sounds for two minutes. Then listen for lung sounds for another three minutes. Overkill feels like an inappropriate word, but five minutes is an extraordinarily long time when you're standing motionless under brilliant white light, your stethoscope pressed against a definitely dead man's chest, observed by his grieving wife. This is why we try and get them out of the room for this bit.

I understand why we take the time to make sure – it's kind of a deal-breaker with death.* The almost-widow keeps asking if I am OK – I don't know whether she thinks I'm too upset to move or have just forgotten what to do next in the death-pronouncing – but every time she says something I leap up like . . . well, like a doctor hearing a noise while listening carefully to the chest of a corpse.

Once I peel myself off the ceiling and compose myself, I confirm the sad news to her and document my findings. It was certainly an agonizing five minutes, but if the whole medicine thing goes tits-up, I'm only a tin of silver Dulux and an old crate away from a gig in Covent Garden as a 'living statue'.

---

* When a Pope dies, zero chances are taken. According to the Vatican's rules, clearly drawn up by someone who thought *The Exorcist* was on the tame side, the doctor has to call out the Pope's name three times, check the body's breath doesn't blow out a candle, then, just to be certain, bop him on the head with a hammer. At least she didn't have to watch me do that.

Tuesday, 5 July 2005

Trying to work out a seventy-year-old lady's alcohol consumption to record in the notes. I've established that wine is her poison.

Me: 'And how much wine do you drink per day, would you say?'

Patient: 'About three bottles on a good day.'

Me: 'OK . . . And on a bad day?'

Patient: 'On a bad day I only manage one.'

Thursday, 7 July 2005

Terrorist atrocities across London, major incident declared, all doctors told to report to A&E.

My responsibility was to go round the surgical wards and discharge any patient whose life or limb wasn't in immediate danger, to clear the decks for new arrivals from the bombings. I was like a snowplough with a stethoscope – booting out anyone who got to the third syllable of 'malingerer' without passing out or coughing up blood. Got rid of hundreds of the bed-blocking fuckers.

Wednesday, 13 July 2005

The hospital didn't receive any casualties, and with no patients I've basically done no work for a week.

Saturday, 23 July 2005

This weekend is my best mate Ron's stag do, and I've had to bail out with barely four hours' notice. It's annoying for a million reasons, from the fact it was just a close selection of pals with only eight of us making the cut, to the personalized T-shirts, to the now-uneven paintballing teams, to the fact I spent four hundred fucking pounds on it.

I was originally due to be working, but arranged a four-way swap (A doing my shift, B doing A's shift, C doing B's shift and me doing C's shift) – so it was always slightly precarious, like a house purchase in a massive chain. And now C (who I've barely met before) has real or imaginary childcare issues for one of her real or imaginary children, so I'm here on the ward instead of Zorbing, off my tits on tequila.

Non-medics* struggle to understand it doesn't actually help having loads of notice for this kind of thing: more than two months' notice means we don't have the rota yet. I order a bottle of whisky I can't afford – I can virtually hear Elton John saying 'Steady on, let's not go crazy here' – and arrange to have it delivered to Ron's flat on his return, alongside my grovelling apologies. We arrange a stag-do postscript for just the two of us in a fortnight's time – after my run of nights, and after the

---

* There should be a term for non-medics, the medical equivalent of 'lay person' or 'civilian'. Patients, maybe?

three locum shifts I booked in to cover the cost of the weekend I'm now missing.

Friday, 29 July 2005

I spend the entire night shift feeling like water is gushing into the hull of my boat and the only thing on hand to bail it out with is a Sylvanian Family rabbit's contact lens.

Everything I'm bleeped about takes at least fifteen minutes to firefight, and I'm getting called about a new blaze every five minutes, so the sums don't *quite* add up. My SHO and registrar are tied up in a busy A&E, so I prioritize the sickest-sounding patients and manage the expectations of the nurses who call me about anything else.

'I'm really sorry but I've got a load of patients who are much more urgent,' I say. 'Realistically, it'll be about six hours.' Some understand and some react like I've just said, 'Fuck off, I'm in the middle of an *Ally McBeal* box-set binge.' I run from chest pain to sepsis to atrial fibrillation to acute asthma all night, like some kind of medical decathlon, and somehow everyone gets through it alive.

At 8 a.m. one of the night sisters bleeps to tell me I did really well tonight and she thinks I'm a good little doctor. I'm willing to overlook the fact that 'good little doctor' sounds like an Enid Blyton character, because I'm pretty sure it's the first time I've had anything approaching a compliment since I qualified. I don't really know what to say but stutter my thanks. In my confusion, I accidentally sign off with, 'Love you, bye.' It's partly out of exhaustion, partly my brain misfiring because H is normally the only person who says nice things to me, and partly because, in that moment, I genuinely loved her for saying that.

2

Senior House Officer – Post One

By August 2005, I was a senior house officer. I was obviously still extremely junior, having only been a doctor for twelve months, but the word 'senior' had now been chucked into my job title. This was presumably to give patients a bit of confidence in the twenty-five-year-old about to take a scalpel to their abdomen. It was also the little morale boost I needed to stop myself jumping off the hospital roof when I first saw my new rota. It would be pushing it to call it a promotion, though – it happens automatically after a year as a house officer, much like when you get a star on your McDonald's badge. Though I suspect Ronald pays better than NHS trusts do.[*]

I believe it's technically possible to fail the house officer year and be required to repeat it, but I've never actually heard of that happening. By way of context, I count among my friends a house officer who slept with a patient in an on-call room, and another who got

_____

[*] My hourly rate as a first year SHO worked out as £6.60. It's slightly more than McDonald's till staff get, though significantly less than a shift supervisor.

distracted and prescribed penicillin instead of paracetamol to a patient with a penicillin allergy. They both
sailed through it, so Christ knows what you have to do
to actually fail.

Senior house officer is the point at which you decide
what to specialize in. If you choose general practice, you
remain in hospital for a couple of years, doing things
like A&E, general medicine and paediatrics, before
moving to the community and being awarded your
elbow patches and permanently raised eyebrow. If you
choose hospital medicine, there are plenty of different
roads you can stumble blindly down. If you fancy yourself as a surgeon, you can sign up to anything from
colorectal surgery to cardiothoracics, neurosurgery to
orthopaedics. (Orthopaedics is basically reserved for the
med school's rugby team – it's barely more than sawing
and nailing – and I suspect they don't 'sign up' for it so
much as dip their hand in ink and provide a palm print.)

There are the various branches of general medicine
if you don't like getting dirt under your nails, such
as geriatrics,* cardiology, respiratory or dermatology
(which can be a revolting but relatively easy life – you

---

* Geriatrics is now known as 'care of the elderly'. Presumably they
want it to sound less clinical – less like a place where someone might
actually expire, and more like a luxury spa where you can get a
mani-pedi while drinking something bright green from a smoothie-
maker. Some hospitals have rebranded the speciality 'care of the
older patient' or 'care of the older person' – I would suggest the more
appropriate 'care of the inevitable'.

can count the number of times you'd be woken up for a dermatological emergency on the fingers of one scaly, flaky hand). Plus there's a bunch of specialities that aren't quite medicine or surgery, like anaesthetics, radiology or obstetrics and gynaecology.

I chose obs and gynae – or 'brats and twats' as it was charmingly known at my medical school. I'd done my BSc thesis in the field, so I had a little bit of a head start, so long as people only asked me questions about early neonatal outcome in the children of mothers with antiphospholipid syndrome, which somehow they never did. I liked that in obstetrics you end up with twice the number of patients you started with, which is an unusually good batting average compared to other specialties. (I'm looking at you, geriatrics.) I also remembered being told by one of the registrars during my student placement that he'd chosen obs and gynae because it was easy. 'Labour ward is literally four things: caesareans, forceps, ventouse and sewing up the mess you've made.'*

I also liked the fact that it was a blend of medicine

---

* About a quarter of babies in the UK are delivered by caesarean section. Some are planned (elective) procedures for things like twins, breech babies or previous caesareans. The rest are unplanned (emergency) caesareans for failure to progress in labour, fetal distress and various other crises. If the baby gets stuck or distressed in the final furlong of a vaginal delivery then you perform an 'instrumental delivery' using either forceps – metal salad servers – or a ventouse, which is a suction cup attached to a vacuum cleaner. I wish I could say those descriptions were an exaggeration.

and surgery – my house officer jobs had proved I shouldn't really be majoring in either. It would give me a chance to work in infertility clinics and labour wards – what could be a better, more rewarding use of my training than delivering babies and helping couples who couldn't otherwise have them? Of course, the job would be difficult emotionally when things went wrong – not every stork has a happy landing – but unfortunately the depth of the lows is the price you pay for the height of the highs.

There was also the fact that I'd ruled out every other speciality in quick succession. Too depressing. Too difficult. Too boring. Too revolting. Obs and gynae was the only one that excited me, a career I could genuinely look forward to.

In the event, it took me months to actually make up my mind, commit and apply. I think the reason I hesitated was that I hadn't made any significant life decisions since I chose which medical school to go to at the age of eighteen – and even that was mostly because I was impressed with the curly fries in the students' union. Age twenty-five was the first point I actually got to make an active decision in the Choose Your Own Adventure book of my life. I not only had to learn how to make a decision, but also ensure I made the right one.

You decide to pick up the forceps. Turn to page 34.

Monday, 8 August 2005

First week working on labour ward. Called in by the midwife because patient DH was feeling unwell shortly after delivering a healthy baby. Nobody likes a clever dick, but it didn't take Columbo, Jessica Fletcher and the entire occupancy of 221b Baker Street to work out the patient was probably 'feeling unwell' because of the litres of blood cascading unnoticed out of her vagina. I pressed the emergency buzzer, hoped someone a bit more useful would appear and unconvincingly reassured the patient that everything was going to be fine, while she continued to redecorate my legs with her blood volume.

The senior registrar ran in, performed a PV* and removed a piece of placenta that was causing the issue.† Once it was coaxed out, and the patient had a few units of blood replaced, she was absolutely fine.

I went to the changing rooms to get myself some fresh scrub trousers. It's the third time in a week my boxers

---

* PV is a per vagina examination. PR is a per rectum examination, so do always clarify when somebody tells you they work in PR.

† If there's anything left in the uterus after delivery – placenta, amniotic membranes, a Lego Darth Vader – the uterus can't contract back down properly, and this causes bleeding until the offending item is removed.

have been soaked in someone else's blood and I've had no option but to chuck them away and continue the shift commando. At £15 a pop for CKs I think I'm running my job at a loss.

This time it had soaked through further than usual and I found myself washing blood off my cock. I'm not sure which is worse: the realization I could have caught HIV or the knowledge that none of my friends would ever believe *this* is how I got it.

Saturday, 27 August 2005

Accosted by a house officer to come and take a look at a post-surgical patient who hasn't passed urine in the last nine hours.* I tell the house officer that I haven't passed urine in the last *eleven* hours because of people like him wasting my time. His face crumples like a crisp packet in a fat kid's fist and I instantly feel terrible for being mean to him – that was me a few months ago. I slink off to review the patient. The patient indeed has no urine output, but that's because the tubing from her catheter is trapped under the wheel of her bed and her bladder is the size of a space hopper. I stop feeling terrible.

---

* Doctors are obsessed with urine output – though not in the kind of way that would make you rethink going on a second date with them – it's how you tell if the patient has a low blood volume. This is particularly bad after surgery as it could mean they're bleeding somewhere or that their kidneys are rogered, neither of which are great.

Monday, 19 September 2005

First ventouse delivery. I suddenly feel like an obstetrician – it's a pretty notional job title until you can, you know, actually extract a baby. My registrar, Lily, talks me through it gently, but I do it all myself and it feels fucking great.

'Congratulations, you did amazingly well there,' says Lily.

'Thank you!' I reply, then realize she's actually talking to the mum.

Wednesday, 21 September 2005

Signing a stack of letters to GPs after gynae clinic when Ernie, one of the registrars – arrogant but funny with it – strides in to borrow an examination lamp. He peers over my shoulder. 'You're going to get struck off if you write that. Change it to "pus-like" or put a hyphen in there somewhere.'

I look down at the offending phrase. 'She has a pussy discharge.'*

---

* At my next hospital, the gynaecology ward was right next to the holding area they put patients in to await transport home, and the sign on the wall said,
GYNAECOLOGY WARD
DISCHARGE LOUNGE

Wednesday, 16 November 2005

I glance at the notes before reviewing an elderly gynae patient on the ward round.

Good news: physio have finally been to see her.

Bad news: the entry reads, 'Patient too drowsy to assess.'

I pop in. The patient is dead.

Tuesday, 22 November 2005

I've assisted registrars and consultants in fifteen caesareans now. On three or four occasions they've offered to let me operate while they teach me the steps, but on every occasion I've wimped out – I'm now the only SHO of the new cohort not to have lost my virginity, as Ernie is so keen on putting it.

Ernie doesn't give me any option today – he introduces me to the patient as the surgeon who's going to deliver her baby. And so I do. Cherry well and truly popped, and with a live audience. I cut through human skin for the first time, open up a uterus for the first time and deliver a baby abdominally for the first time. I'd like to say it was an amazing experience, but I was concentrating far too hard on every step to actually take any of it in.

The caesarean takes a laborious fifty-five minutes*

---

* An uncomplicated caesarean should only take twenty to twenty-five minutes, with the wind in the right direction.

from start to end, and Ernie is remarkably patient with me. As I clean up the wound afterwards, he points out that my incision was on the wonk by about ten degrees. He says to the patient, 'You'll notice when you take the dressing off that we had to go in at a bit of an angle,' which she somehow seems to accept without question – the miracle of motherhood sugaring that particular pill.

Ernie shows me how to write up the operation notes and debriefs me over coffee, stretching his virginity metaphor to within an inch of its life like he's some kind of sex pervert. Apparently, with practice my technique will improve, it'll get less bloody and less nerve-wracking, and eventually it'll all just start feeling like a boring routine. The anaesthetist chips in: 'I wouldn't try and make your performance last any longer though.'

Thursday, 22 December 2005

Clinical incident. Bleeped at 2 a.m. and asked to review a gynaecology inpatient who was unconscious. I suggest to the nurse that most people are unconscious at 2 a.m., but she is still extremely keen that I attend urgently. The patient's GCS* is 14/15, so 'unconscious' is rather

---

* GCS, or Glasgow Coma Scale, is a measure of conscious level. You get a mark from 1–4 for eye response, 1–5 for verbal response and 1–6 for motor response, giving you a maximum total score of 15 if completely normal and a lowest possible score of 3 if you're dead. (Or a score of 2 if you're dead and have no eyes.) For some reason,

pushing it, but she is disorientated and clearly hypo-glycaemic. A nurse traipses off to find a blood glucose monitor for me from another ward. I'm fairly confident of my diagnosis so decide not to wait, and ask for the bottle of orange squash we keep handy in the clinical fridge for this situation. The patient drinks it but remains drowsy. It's a bit late at night to be playing House, but I order some other tests and try to work out what else could be going on, as we wait for the machine to arrive. There's never one to hand, even though they're required all the time and cost about a tenner in Boots. I was thinking about just buying my own one, but it feels like a slippery slope that ends with keeping an X-ray machine in the back of the car.

The healthcare assistant points out that the empty bottle he was about to throw away is sugar-free orange squash – about as much use in this situation as a book token. I don't know whether to laugh or cry, but am too tired to do either. A couple of nursing desk Ferrero Rochers later and the patient is feeling much better. The

---

as if doctors' lives aren't hard enough already, patients – particularly in A&E – seem to enjoy pretending that they're more unconscious than they actually are. In this situation, the textbooks teach applying a painful stimulus to assess if they're faking it, such as pressing hard on a fingernail or rubbing your knuckles on their breastbone. My preferred method was always to raise one of their arms up and drop it onto their face. If they're faking, they don't let their arm plomp onto their face and it miraculously floats off to one side. The down-side is if they're genuinely unconscious and you have to explain yourself to their relatives.

nurse in charge apologizes for an 'ordering error' and promises they'll stock the right kind in future. Two quid says next time I see a hypoglycaemic patient they nip off to the fridge and return holding a butternut squash.

Sunday, 25 December 2005

Good news/Bad news.

Good news: it's Christmas morning.*

Bad news: I have to work on labour ward.

Worse news: my phone goes off. It's my registrar. I didn't set my alarm and now they're wondering where the hell I am.

Even worse news: I'm asleep in my car. It takes me a while to establish where I am or why.

Good news: it seems I fell asleep after my shift last night and I'm already at work, in the hospital car park.

I leap out of the car, grab a quick shower and then I'm good to go, a mere ten minutes late. I have eight missed

---

* In the NHS, it's irrelevant that you worked the Christmas before, firstly because that was almost certainly in a different hospital and, secondly, nobody gives the tiniest toss. There's a pecking order of those least likely to work at Christmas: first up is the doctor who organizes the rota, followed by those with kids. Several rungs further down this hierarchy came me, my childlessness lumbering me with Christmas shifts practically every year. Despite no great paternal yearnings (a feeling exacerbated by working on labour ward), I seriously considered *pretending* to have children when I started a new job.

calls from H and a text saying 'Merry Christmas', full stop, no kiss.

This year we're doing Christmas on my next day off: the sixth of January. 'Just think how reduced the crackers will be by then!' was the only positive I could offer.

Wednesday, 18 January 2006

There are days when you get firm confirmation of your place in the hospital hierarchy, and today's leveller was a cord prolapse.[*]

I clamber onto the mattress behind the patient and assume the veterinary position, and the bed gets wheeled through to theatre. Another caesarean is just finishing off, so we wait in the anaesthetic room for the time being. To keep the patient calm and make the situation seem less weird, we have a mundane chat about baby names, nappies and maternity leave.

---

[*] Cord prolapse means that a loop or two of umbilical cord comes out through the vagina during labour, and unless this is right at the point of delivery, it means a very urgent caesarean. Fair enough that the cord got a little caught up in the moment and couldn't wait to make an appearance, like a firework exploding on the fourth of November, but if it gets cold it goes into spasm, meaning there'll be no blood going to baby. So, it needs to be popped back into the vagina, and to keep pressure off the cord, the mother has to go up on all fours, resting on her knees and elbows, with the doctor standing behind until the moment she gets laid on her back for the caesarean. The doctor wears a very long glove that goes right up to the shoulder and is revoltingly called 'The Gauntlet'.

Her partner had nipped to the cafe downstairs for a few minutes just before things got this . . . intimate, so he missed all the drama. On his return, the midwife quickly brings him up to speed and gets him changed into scrubs so he can come to theatre for the caesarean. She leads him into the anaesthetic room, where I'm kneeling, the vulva of the mother of his child halfway up my forearm. 'Jesus Christ!' he says, in a heavy Glasgow accent. The midwife remonstrates that she'd warned him I'd be holding the cord out of the way. 'You did,' he says, his eyes like dinner plates. 'You didn't say he'd be wearing her like Sooty though.'

Tuesday, 24 January 2006

God has had the good sense to stay the hell away from my job, aside from a few 'Holy fuck's and the odd 'Jesus!'. Today I meet MM, a Jehovah's Witness, to consent her for an open myomectomy.* It's a bloody type of operation, and we should have four units of cross-matched blood in the theatre fridge on standby.

The snag is, of course, that Jehovah's Witnesses refuse any blood transfusions because of their (fucking stupid) belief that blood contains the soul, and you shouldn't put someone else's soul into you. Nonetheless,

---

* A myomectomy is the removal of fibroids – benign swirls of growth in the muscle of the uterus that you remove using what is essentially a corkscrew.

it's a free country – so we respect everyone's (fucking stupid) values and wishes.

MM is bright, charming and erudite, and we have a very interesting discussion. She agrees to have cell salvage* performed during the operation and I give her the specific consent form for refusing blood transfusion, even if needed to save her life. A small possibility but a real one, even with cell salvage – numerous Jehovah's Witnesses have died because they declined blood products. She signs, though admits part of the reason is that her family would never speak to her again if she received blood. (Even more of an incentive to have a transfusion if you ask me.)

Mr Flitwick, my consultant, tells me that in his sepia-tinted, gung-ho version of 'the good old days' they'd just ignore the form and plough ahead with a blood transfusion regardless, if needed – the patient would never find out as they'd be under anaesthetic. Happily, today's operation is gloriously uneventful and the cell salvage machine stays in the corner of the room. I review her back on the ward in the evening and on leafing through

---

* Cell salvage involves hoovering up any blood that's lost during the operation, rather than swabbing it away, then running it through a machine that filters out any impurities (water used during the procedure, surgeon's sweat, bits of paint that have flaked off the ceiling). Should there be any need for a transfusion, the patient's own blood can be returned to them – and some Witnesses are happy this is in accordance with their teachings, as the blood stays within a closed circuit and isn't thought to have truly left the body. I know.

her notes I see that her birthday is in two days' time and she'll most likely still be in hospital. I commiserate, despite the fact that I, too, will very likely be in a hospital for every single one of my birthdays until I'm too weak to blow out the candles, but she tells me that Jehovah's Witnesses don't celebrate birthdays or even receive presents. This is even more fucked-up than the whole blood thing.

Thursday, 26 January 2006

Moral maze. On the ward round, Ernie is talking to a very well-spoken woman in her thirties – basically a younger, posher version of the Queen. She's now ready to go home, after an emergency admission a few days ago with ovarian torsion.* He books her in for review in outpatients in six weeks and tells her not to drive for three weeks. 'Oh, for heaven's sake!' she says to Ernie. 'The bloody thing's in the car park here. Why don't you just drive it until I see you in clinic?' Ernie is about to say no, that's insane, until she complicates matters by pulling a set of Bentley keys from her handbag. Anyway, Ernie currently drives a Bentley Continental GT.

---

* Ovarian torsion is where the ovary twists round on itself and cuts off its blood supply – if not operated on very quickly, it goes black and dies. And if not operated on at all, the entire patient becomes septic, then goes black and dies.

Friday, 27 January 2006

I've been visiting Baby L on SCBU* for three months now – it's become part of my routine before I head home, and it's nice to see a familiar face, even if it's through the glass of an incubator wall.† His mum was admitted on my second Saturday in the job, twenty-six weeks into her first pregnancy, with a blistering head-ache that it quickly transpired was severe early onset pre-eclampsia.‡ She was stabilized and we delivered Baby L on the Sunday; I assisted the consultant in the

---

* SCBU (pronounced Scaboo) is the Special Care Baby Unit, NICU is Neonatal Intensive Care, PICU is Paediatric Intensive Care, PIKACHU is a type of Pokémon.

† Something very unsatisfying about house-officer jobs was the way you never found out the end of the story – every patient's box set was missing the final DVD. A patient would come in with pneumonia, you'd get him well enough to go home, and then he's gone – he could live another fifteen years, die on the bus home or anything in between and you'd almost certainly never know. Extreme nosiness aside, it always felt like it might have been useful to find out if our manage-ment plans were any use. I liked that obstetrics played out much quicker – you would get to watch right through to the credits; and by reflecting back on your decisions in the context of these outcomes, you could learn and improve as a doctor. And so, if a baby went to SCBU, I made a point of popping by to see how they were doing.

‡ Pre-eclampsia is a disorder of pregnancy which can affect most organs of the mum's body, causing liver and kidney damage, swelling of the brain, fluid in the lungs and platelet problems, as well as problems with baby's growth and well-being. It ultimately progresses to eclampsia – life-threatening fits. Most cases of pre-eclampsia are mild, but every pregnant patient has their blood pressure and urine protein measured at each visit, in order to pick up the condition at

45

section. Mum ended up spending a few days in intensive care – so we definitely couldn't have waited any longer before delivering – and baby came out a tiny scrap of a thing, weighing in at just over a jar of jam.

Neonatologists make obstetricians look like orthopaedic surgeons – they're so academic, so meticulous – defying God and nature to make these babies pull through. As recently as 1970, this baby would have had chances of survival under 10 per cent, but today the odds are over 90 per cent. After twelve weeks of neonatal magic he's gone from a transparent-skinned shrew attached to a dozen tubes and wires to a proper screaming, vomiting, sleeping little baby, and he's getting discharged home this afternoon.

I should be delighted he's going home – and I am, of course, that's our entire raison d'être – but I'm going to miss seeing my little pal every couple of days.

I buy the least ghastly card they have in the League of Friends shop and leave it with the paediatric nurses to pass on to his mum. I say how pleased I am their story had a happy ending, give her my phone number and ask her to maybe text me a picture of him every so

---

an early stage. The only cure for pre-eclampsia is delivering the placenta (and necessarily the baby first). For the vast majority of pre-eclamptic patients, they'll end up just being monitored throughout pregnancy, taking some tablets to reduce their blood pressure or having labour induced a week or two early. Some patients, however, develop the condition severely and much earlier in pregnancy, leading to the painful decision to deliver the baby prematurely, to prevent terrible consequences for both mother and child.

often. Yes, it's probably against GMC regulations and hospital protocol and contravenes all sorts of small print, guidelines and best practice, but I'm prepared to go down for this one.*

Thursday, 2 February 2006

Signing letters to GPs in the gynae office.

> *Dear Doctor,*
>
> *I saw XA in clinic with her husband Sam, Esther Sugar and their two children . . .*

A moment while I try to remember the appointment. Who of these three were the children's parents? I feel I should know who Esther is – why the full name? Is she famous? Wife of Sir Alan? As it turns out, Esther wasn't there at all.

Two months ago, the trust laid off almost all the hospital secretaries, replacing them with a new computer system. The first key difference is that rather than giving your Dictaphone tapes to the secretaries, you now dictate straight onto your clinic computer, which chooses to either upload your audio and send it abroad to the secretarial equivalent of a sweatshop or to instantly delete it without trace. The second key difference is that the quality of the transcription would suggest the back-end of the system involves two tin cans, a length of string

---

* And she did text me.

47

and a lemur who's been trained to type. We're not to worry about that though: the main thing is all the money the trust is saving by sacking so many long-serving, hard-working members of staff who adored the hospital. The one advantage of this system is that you can listen back to your original audio when reviewing documents. I press play.

'Dear Doctor,

I saw XA in clinic with her husband Sam (S for sugar) and their two children.'

I'm confident this takes me to the top of the leader board in departmental dictation fuck-ups, unseating 'The patient has known analogies' (no known allergies).

Wednesday, 22 March 2006

Three a.m. attendance at labour ward triage. Patient RO is twenty-five years old and thirty weeks into her first pregnancy. She complains of a large number of painless spots on her tongue. Diagnosis: taste buds.

Monday, 3 April 2006

It's 2 a.m. and there's not much doing on labour ward so I slope off to the on-call room to catch up on some personal admin (Adamin?) and stare at Facebook for a bit. I comment on how cute a friend's latest ugly baby looks, which I can do very convincingly as I spend a large proportion of my working day doing the same thing to total strangers. For me, the true miracle of childbirth is that smart, rational people with jobs and the ability to vote look at these half-melted fleshy blobs, their heads misshapen from being squeezed through a pelvis, covered in five types of horrendous gunk, looking like they've spent a good two hours rolling around on top of a deep-pan pizza, and honestly believe they look beautiful. It's Darwinism in action, an irrational love for your progeny. The same hardwired desire to keep the species going that sees them come back to labour ward for round two, eighteen months after the irreparable destruction of their perineum.

The other miracle of childbirth is that I can put metal forceps on a baby's head and lean backwards – applying 20 kg of traction force on it, generally getting a sweat on – and the baby comes out absolutely fine, rather than, as you might expect, decapitated. Once it's born, every new mother obsesses over keeping the head straight with a cradled hand. If photographs could talk, 'Careful of his neck!' is the shriek you'd hear over any picture of a childless relative posing with a newborn. But I'm pretty sure you could carry it by its head and it'd be totally OK.*

I'm just going through exes' profiles to check they're colossally miserable and overweight without me when I see a post pop up from Simon, a school friend's younger brother. He's twenty-two and even though I've only

---

* This is not medical advice.

spoken to him twice, a decade ago, this is Facebook, where everyone's your friend. It's simple and devastatingly effective. Four words: 'Goodbye everyone. I'm done.'

I realize I'm probably the only person to be reading this at 2.30 a.m. on a Monday, so I send him a private message to ask if he's OK. I say I'm awake, remind him I'm a doctor and give him my mobile number. I'm scrolling through my phone to see if I have his brother's number, when Simon rings. He's an absolute mess: drunk, crying. He's just split up with his girlfriend.

I'm actually no better trained to counsel him than I would be to talk him through replacing a gearbox or laying a parquet floor, but he assumes I am, and that's good enough for both of us. Two (miraculously bleep-free) hours later and we've had a good chat. He's going to get a cab to his mum's then make an emergency appointment with his GP in the morning. I feel the same weird endorphin rush as after dealing with any medical emergency – exhaustion plus exhilaration and the vague feeling of having done a 'good thing' (like how you'd feel after running a 10k for charity). It's likely I've made a bigger difference to Simon than any of my patients tonight.

I answer a bleep and head to labour ward to review a woman at thirty weeks who decided she needed her eczema seen at 5 a.m. 'I thought it would be quieter now than in the morning,' she says.

Monday, 10 April 2006

Referral from an A&E SHO – patient has some kind of warty vulval growth. I ask him if he can describe it a bit more. 'Like cauliflower florets, mate. Actually, what with the discharge, it's more like broccoli.'

H did not enjoy this story over dinner.

Friday, 21 April 2006

Ron is having a minor knee op next week and wants me to reassure him that he's not going to die during the anaesthetic, reassurance that I'm underqualified yet perfectly happy to give him.

He also asks if sometimes the anaesthetic 'doesn't work', so I tell him a story from earlier this year at work:

'So, there are two main drugs that anaesthetists give. Firstly, a muscle relaxant – so that the surgeon can have a proper fiddle around. With the body completely paralysed, you can't breathe unassisted, which is why you get hooked up to a ventilator during the procedure. The second drug's a cloudy fluid called propofol, which makes you unconscious, so you're asleep throughout the procedure.*

'Now imagine that your anaesthetist accidentally grabs the wrong cloudy fluid off his trolley and injects

---

* Or indefinitely if you're Michael Jackson.

51

you with an antibiotic instead of propofol. You're lying on an anaesthetic table, totally paralysed by a muscle relaxant, but without the propofol you're entirely awake – able to hear everything that's being said, able to feel the surgeon cleaning you up with antiseptic and with no way of alerting anyone that something's gone horribly wrong. You silently scream as his scalpel cuts through your skin – a worse, more searing pain than you've ever experienced in your life . . .' Ron's expression looks like it's been drawn on by Edvard Munch. 'But I'm sure you'll be just fine!'

Tuesday, 6 June 2006

Called to see a patient in A&E. She had a Medical Termination of Pregnancy a couple of days ago and is in absolute agony. I don't quite know what the matter is, but something is definitely up – I admit her to the ward for pain relief and senior review. Ernie examines her.

'She's having cramping pains. Scan before her MTOP showed an intrauterine pregnancy. Normal. Send her home.'

I try to justify my admission – surely this is way too much pain? She's on morphine!

'Only because you prescribed her morphine . . .'

No one is in pain like this with an MTOP, though.

'How do *you* know her pain threshold?' comes the no-nonsense reply. 'Maybe she's like this when she stubs her toe as well.'

I venture that something weird is going on here, and he dismisses me.

'If you hear hooves clip-clopping outside your bedroom window, it *could* be a zebra. But when you take a look, it will almost always turn out to be a horse.' He tells me I can prescribe her some antibiotics just in case there's an infection brewing – but she still needs to go home.

The bleep from the ward saying that the patient had deteriorated would ideally have come at that exact moment. Instead, it came a few hours later, but the result was the same: assisting Ernie in theatre to remove an ectopic pregnancy* and a metric fuck-tonne of blood from her pelvis. The scan she'd had before her termination was dangerously wrong.

The patient is now fine and back on the ward. Ernie hasn't apologized to me, as that would require him to change his entire personality. I'm currently on Amazon, ordering him a key ring in the shape of a zebra.

---

* An ectopic pregnancy is when an embryo attaches in the wrong place – most frequently in a fallopian tube. Left untreated, they will eventually rupture, and this is the most common cause of death in women in the first three months of pregnancy. Every woman with pain and a positive pregnancy test must be considered as having an ectopic unless otherwise proven by a scan. In this case, the scanner had mistakenly interpreted an ectopic pregnancy as an intrauterine one.

Monday, 12 June 2006

Counselling a patient that weight loss would help control her PCOS,* I refer her to the dietician and ask her about exercise. Just because something is obvious to me, it might not always be obvious to the patient – it feels like knocking on the door of a blazing building to tell the owner their house is on fire, but occasionally it does make a difference. Steeling myself for the predictable answer about a lack of time, I offer: 'It might help you to join a gym?'

'I'm a member of one already,' comes the reply. 'But I haven't been in about £3,000.'

Monday, 19 June 2006

Called to urgently review an antenatal patient on the ward. Patient ES has begun induction of labour for post-maturity.† The concerned midwife leads me to a toilet

---

* Polycystic Ovarian Syndrome (PCOS) is the most common endocrine condition in women, affecting between 1 in 5 and 1 in 20 females, depending on how they define it, which will have changed another three or four times between me writing this and anyone reading it. PCOS can cause problems with fertility, skin and body hair, and menstrual disturbance.

† Much like your drunk mate insisting you go on to one more club even though she's already got vomit in her hair, pregnancies sometimes keep going longer than is wise. After forty-two weeks the placenta can start to give up the ghost, so we induce labour before mums get to that point, the first step being a vaginal pessary such as Prostin.

on the ward; the patient has just opened her bowels and the pan looks like Lush have released a horrific new red and brown bath bomb. It doesn't augur well for either the cleaners' tea break or the patient herself.

I examine her to check the bleeding isn't vaginal, which it isn't, and am pleased to see the baby looks fine on the CTG.* The rectal examination was totally normal, the patient says she's never had anything like this before and has no other symptoms. I send off bloods, crossmatch her, put up some fluids and refer her urgently to gastro. I also google whether Prostin can cause massive gastrointestinal bleeding. There's no history of it happening before, so this would be the first case – I idly wonder whether they'll name the syndrome after me. I was rather hoping Kay Syndrome might be a more glamorous discovery than someone shitting themselves inside out during induction of labour, but perhaps it's a price worth paying for immortalization in the textbooks.

The gastro consultant appears before I've finished writing up my notes, and after a quick chat and another lubricated finger, she's wheeled off for a colonoscopy. Happily, all looks normal and there's no evidence of recent bleeding. A bit of further questioning and the

---

* The cardiotocograph, known as the CTG or 'trace', is a belt strapped to mums during labour that measures and continuously records a tracing of contractions and baby's heart rate. They are generally described as a 'reassuring trace' or a 'non-reassuring trace'.

consultant comes up with the diagnosis: he bleeps to let me know.

The nightmare in the toilet bowl I'd witnessed was in fact the rather damning evidence of the two large jars of pickled beetroot that ES had inexplicably taken it upon herself to eat the night before. Next time I want to refer him someone's bowel movement, the consultant 'respectfully' asks that I taste it first.

Tuesday, 20 June 2006

Our computer system has been upgraded and, as happens eleven times out of ten when the hospital tries to make life easier, they've made everything much more complicated. It certainly looks much whizzier (and less like an MS-DOS program from school), but they've not actually fixed any of the massive clunking problems with the software, they've just slapped an interface on top of it. It's the equivalent of treating skin cancer by putting make-up over the lesion. Actually, it's worse than that. This glossy interface uses so much of the exhausted system's resources that it's now slowed to a nearly unusable crawl. It's like treating skin cancer with some make-up that the patient has an extreme allergic reaction to.

The blood tests now all live in a drop-down menu, and to order one involves scrolling down an alphabetical list of every test any doctor has ever ordered in the history of humanity. To get down to 'Vitamin B12' takes 3 minutes 17 seconds. And if you press the letter 'V' rather than wading down there manually, then the system crashes so badly you have to turn the computer off at the wall and all but use a soldering iron to get it working again. Ninety-nine per cent of the time we order the same dozen tests and yet, rather than prioritizing those at the top of the list (even the easyJet website knows to put the UK above Albania and Azerbaijan), they're scattered throughout a billion tests I've never heard of or requested. Who knew there were three different lab tests for serum selenium? As a result, there's a very narrow window of anaemic patients I will now order Vitamin B12 levels for. If you're only mildly anaemic I'm not wasting the day with my finger pressing on the down arrow for three minutes. And if you're severely anaemic, I won't order it because you'll probably be dead by the time I've done so.

Friday, 21 July 2006

Bleeped to the gynae ward at 5 a.m. to write a discharge summary for a patient due to go home in the morning. It should have been done during the day by her own SHO and there's no reason for me to be doing it. But if I don't do it tonight then it will delay the patient's discharge. I sit down and get on with it – it's fairly mindless work so gives me a bit of time to plot some appropriate revenge act on the SHO in question. On my way out, I notice the light is on in patient CR's side room, so I pop my head in to check if everything's OK.

I admitted her from A&E last week with tense asci-tes* and the suspicion of an ovarian mass. I've been on nights since and not caught up with what's happened. She tells me. Suspicion of an ovarian mass has become a diagnosis of ovarian cancer has become confirmation of widespread metastases has become talk of a few months left. When I saw her in A&E, despite obvious suspicions, I didn't say the word 'cancer' – I was taught that if you say the word even in passing, that's all a patient remembers. Doesn't matter what else you do, utter the C-word just once and you've basically walked into the cubicle and said nothing but 'cancer cancer cancer cancer cancer' for half an hour. And not that you'd ever want a patient to have cancer of course, I really *really* didn't want her to. Friendly, funny, chatty – despite the litres of fluid in her abdomen splinting her breathing – we were like two long-lost pals finding themselves next to each other at a bus stop and catching up on all our years apart. Her son has a place at med school, her daughter is at the same school my sister went to, she recognized my socks were Duchamp. I stuck in a Bonanno catheter to take off the fluid and admitted her to the ward for the day team to investigate.

And now she's telling me what they found. She bursts into tears, and out come all the 'will never's, the crushing realization that 'forever' is just a word on the front of Valentine's cards. Her son will qualify from medical

---

* Ascites is fluid in the abdomen, and almost always very bad news.

school – she won't be there. Her daughter will get married – she won't be able to help with the table plan or throw confetti. She'll never meet her grandchildren. Her husband will never get over it. 'He doesn't even know how to work the thermostat!' She laughs, so I laugh. I really don't know what to say. I want to lie and tell her everything's going to be fine, but we both know that it won't. I hug her. I've never hugged a patient before – in fact, I think I've only hugged a grand total of five people, and one of my parents isn't on that list – but I don't know what else to do.

We talk about boring practical things, rational concerns, irrational concerns, and I can see from her eyes it's helping her. It suddenly strikes me that I'm almost certainly the first person she's opened up to about all this, the only one she's been totally honest with. It's a strange privilege, an honour I didn't ask for.

The other thing I realize is that none of her many, many concerns are about herself; it's all about the kids, her husband, her sister, her friends. Maybe that's the definition of a good person.

We had a patient in obstetrics a couple of months ago who was diagnosed with metastatic breast cancer during pregnancy, and was advised to deliver at thirty-two weeks so she could start treatment, but waited until thirty-seven weeks to give her baby the absolute best possible chance. She died after a fortnight spent with her baby – who knows whether starting treatment a month sooner would have made any difference. Probably not.

And now I'm sitting with a woman who's asking me if she shouldn't have her ashes scattered on the Scilly Isles. It's her favourite spot, but she doesn't want it to be a sad place for her family once she's gone. The undiluted selflessness of someone fully aware what her absence will do to those she leaves behind. My bleep goes off – it's the morning SHO asking for handover. I've spent two hours in this room, the longest I've ever spent with a patient who wasn't under anaesthetic. On the way home I phone my mum to tell her I love her.

3

Senior House Officer – Post Two

Sometime during my early years as an SHO, I remember watching a documentary about Shaolin grandmasters. They train for a decade or more in a remote temple, waking up at 5 a.m. and only stopping at midnight, submitting themselves to a life of celibacy, devoid of material possessions. I couldn't help but feel it didn't sound that bad – at least they didn't have to uproot their lives every year to a completely different temple.

NHS deaneries, who are responsible for postgraduate medical training, move doctors to different hospitals every six or twelve months to ensure they learn from a broad range of consultants, which I guess makes sense. Unfortunately, each deanery covers a fairly large geo-graphical area, and you get randomly allocated to units throughout that region. For example, one such deanery is Kent, Surrey and Sussex: which I (and indeed the Ordnance Survey) had always considered to be three enormous, separate areas. Another deanery is Scotland. You know Scotland, that – what would you call it, oh yes – entire *country* measuring over 30,000 square miles. If you're deciding where to buy your first house, it's rather difficult to choose a location that's handy for all of Scotland. Even if you were insane enough to put yourself through a property transaction once or twice a year, it would be fairly tricky as the deaneries limit relocation costs to a princely zero pounds.

So while all my friends in sensible careers were getting mortgages and puppies, H and I were taking on year-long rental contracts and living somewhere mutually inconvenient roughly halfway between our two workplaces. It was yet another item on the list of ways my job was inflicting collateral damage on H – medical widow, post-shift counsellor and now nomad.

I remember once phoning round all the various utilities and DVLA and so on about our change of address (I think as penance because I couldn't take the day off work to help with the move) and the home insurance people asked a standard question about the number of nights the property is left empty. I realized that if I lived alone, the policy would be invalid as it would technically be considered an 'unoccupied property'.

Despite the hours, I'd really enjoyed my first year in obs and gynae – I'd made the right choice. I'd gone from a tottering Bambi, terrified every time the bleep went off, to, if not a graceful roebuck, then at least someone who could do a decent impression of one. I now had a bit of self-belief that I could deal with the emergency behind each delivery-room door; mostly thanks to working in a hospital with seniors who were invested in my development as a doctor.

When the deanery rolled their dice for the second time, however, I found myself in a much more old-fashioned hospital. If you describe a grandparent as being 'old-fashioned', it's a euphemism for 'talks about ordering a Chinky'. In a hospital setting, it means 'unsupportive'. You're on your own.

I'd gone from a nursery slope straight to a Schumacher-splattering black run, where they took the now largely extinct approach of 'see one, do one, teach one'. You've watched someone remove a fallopian tube or scan an ovary, so that's you fully trained up. You'd be forgiven for thinking this was a horrible nightmare. As it turned out at this hospital, it was often the best-case scenario, 'see one' frequently getting skipped over, like foreplay in a nightclub toilet tryst.

Nowadays, YouTube instructional videos can show you anything from how to repair an ingrown toenail to separating conjoined twins.* Back in 2006, you had to follow a list of printed instructions in a textbook. To add to the fun, you'd have to memorize these generally quite complicated steps (think kit car rather than IKEA wardrobe) before you saw the patient. How much confidence would you have in someone staring into your genitals with a scalpel in one hand and a manual in the other? I rapidly learned to maintain an air of absolute confidence, no matter how frantically my legs were paddling under the water. In summary, never play poker

---

* Please don't attempt either.

with me. Although do bear me in mind if you're struggling with your flat-pack furniture.

Because I spent the vast proportion of my waking hours at work and because the deep end was so very deep, I learned a lot during my second SHO post and did so very quickly. The 'old-fashioned' method might not be any fun, but it definitely works. Those Shaolin bastards were basically at holiday camp.

Wednesday, 2 August 2006

It's Black Wednesday[*] and I have started at St Agatha's. It is an established fact that death rates go up on Black Wednesday. Knowing this really takes the pressure off, so I'm not trying very hard.

Thursday, 10 August 2006

Reviewing a mother in clinic, six weeks after a traumatic delivery. All is now well, but something is clearly troubling her. I ask her what's up and she breaks down in tears – she thinks the baby has a brain tumour and asks me to have a look. It's very much not my department[†] but one look at the mother's collapsed face tells me that now perhaps wouldn't be the best time to play the unhelpful station assistant at a ticket window and advise

---

[*] All junior doctors change hospitals on exactly the same day every six or twelve months, which is known as Black Wednesday. You might think it would be a terrible idea to exchange all your Scrabble tiles in one go and expect the hospital to run exactly as it did the day before, and you'd be quite right.

[†] Parents seem to think obstetricians are wise owls with expert knowledge of infants, but this couldn't be further from the truth. We know the square root of fuck all about them, save for a few half-remembered semi-facts from medical school. Once a baby's no longer umbilically attached to its mother, we hand them over and never deal with them again until they're old enough to procreate.

65

she should see her GP. I examine the child and hope that whatever she's concerned about is within the limited parameters of my paediatric knowledge.

She shows me a hard swelling on the back of baby's head. My ship has somehow come in and I can confidently announce that this is baby's occipital protuberance, which is a completely normal part of the skull. Look, there it is on your other kid's head! There it is on your head!

'Oh my God,' she cries, the tears still streaking her face, eyes darting from her baby to her three-year-old and back again, like she's watching Wimbledon. 'It's hereditary.'

Monday, 14 August 2006

My rota involves scanning in the Early Pregnancy Unit once a fortnight. Today, having never so much as *seen* a scan like this performed before, I had to single-shaking-handedly run a clinic of twenty patients, peering at 4 mm lumps of cells using a trans-vaginal probe.*

I asked (begged) a registrar to give me a quick demo, and he had time to see one patient with me before he dashed off to theatre. My SHO colleague on the after-

---

* This sounds like a high-speed train service in the Caucasus but is considerably less sophisticated. You look inside with an ultrasound stick to decide if a pregnancy is viable, miscarrying or ectopic. Misdiagnosis can see you the wrong side of a negligence/manslaughter charge.

noon shift had never done it before either, so I passed on my new skill by scanning her first patient for her. See one, do twenty, teach one.

Wednesday, 16 August 2006

Just out of a delivery, my slickest ventouse yet. The midwife told me afterwards she assumed I was a registrar (although she *is* known as Dangerous Dawn, so I'm not going to put vast quantities of stock in that).

A phone call from Mum to say my sister Sophie's got into med school. I send Soph a text with huge congratulations, then a picture of me thumbs-upping in scrubs (cropped above the splatter-zone) and 'You in six years' time!'

Had the call come at the end of the shift, my text would have read, 'RUN LIKE THE FUCKING WIND.'

Monday, 21 August 2006

I've been carrying a Post Office 'Sorry you were out' card around with me for over a fortnight. I keep taking it out and looking at it meaningfully like it's a photograph of my firstborn or some long-dead childhood sweetheart, pathetically rereading the collection office's opening times in the hope they will magically alter before my eyes. They do not.

I wouldn't have time to get to the Post Office and back in my lunch hour, even if I had a lunch hour, which of course I don't, but I've been holding on to a glimmer of hope that I might knock off work early one day – if the hospital burnt down, say, or nuclear war was declared. Today I start a week of nights so nip off to collect the parcel. Unfortunately, it turns out the Post Office only hold on to items for eighteen days, every one of which I've been at work, so it's been returned to sender.

Long story short, H won't be getting a birthday present tomorrow.

Thursday, 14 September 2006

Patient CW on the antenatal ward needs some imaging done of her lungs, so I book her in for an MRI and go through the checklist.* She is in fact ineligible for an MRI, having had a small but powerful magnet implanted in the pulp of her right index finger a few years ago.

---

* Ordinarily you'd do a CT scan, but we try to avoid those in pregnancy as they involve a large quantity of X-ray exposure; and anyone who's stayed up for the late-night horror can tell you that radiation plus baby is not a good idea. I've had the mechanism of MRIs explained to me any number of times and I'm still none the wiser, but no X-rays are involved: images are obtained using a combination of protons, magic and an enormous fucking magnet. And I mean enormous; the size and weight of a one-bedroom flat. The MRI checklist asks if they've got a metal heart valve (it would tear out of their now-dead chest at 80 mph and splat onto the machine) or worked in a metal factory (tiny bits of metal would have found their way into their eyes, making both eyeballs explode upon opening the door to the MRI suite).

Apparently there had been a limited trend for this, performed by tattoo artists and intended to give the recipient an 'extra sense' – an other-worldly awareness of metal objects around them, like a kind of vibrating aura (her words) or a slightly low-rent X-Man (my words).

Her sales pitch needs work, to be honest. It turned out not to be the mystical, ethereal experience she had been looking for, but a regal pain in the arse – she tells me it's become infected a number of times and going through airport security is now a living hell. I briefly toy with asking her to brush past my colleague Cormac to either confirm or refute the rumour that he has a Prince Albert,* but she says the implant has recently become either dislodged or demagnetized and she now barely feels a thing, except for a lump in her finger. She wants to have the magnet removed, in fact, but the scar tissue that will have formed around it makes it a slightly involved operation, and one not covered on the NHS. I book her in for a CT scan – she can wear a lead apron and there'll be very little radiation exposure for the baby. Although if I'd only gone ahead and booked her an MRI, I'd have saved her the cost of that private operation.

---

* The already close-to-zero appeal of a genital piercing instantly evaporated as a house officer when I saw a patient present with a ring that had ripped out during sex. This happens frequently enough that urologists have a term for it: 'Prince Albert's revenge'.

Sunday, 17 September 2006

Either the printer has gone insane or one of the receptionists has – huge quantities of paper have engulfed the nursing station. Everyone in sight has collected around to try and fix it, all doing exactly the same thing – jabbing random buttons to absolutely zero effect.

Pages are cascading out of the printer and onto the labour ward floor. I pick one up – they're patient identification stickers for a neonate, to go on notes, wristbands, etc. For the rest of the day, everyone checks their shoes and backs in paranoia, just in case a stray one has become attached – this is one label nobody wants to be walking around with. A slightly unfortunate surname means that every sticker says BABY RAPER.

Monday, 25 September 2006

How the other half live. In antenatal clinic, an extremely posh patient attends for a routine appointment. All is well with her extremely posh fetus. Her extremely posh eight-year-old asks her a question about the economy (!), and before she answers she asks her extremely posh five-year-old, 'Do you know what the economy is, darling?'

'Yes, Mummy. It's the part of the plane that's terrible.'

You can see how revolutions start.

I'm off sick for the first time since qualifying. Work weren't exactly sympathetic.

'Oh, for fuck's sake,' spat my registrar when I rang in. 'Can't you just come in for the morning?' I explained I had quite bad food poisoning and was in some kind of gastrointestinal meltdown. 'Fine,' he said with the kind of weary, simmering passive-aggression I normally only get at home. 'But phone around and find someone who's on leave to cover you.'

I'm pretty sure this isn't the protocol at Google or GlaxoSmithKline or even Ginsters. Is there a single other workplace where you'd conceivably be asked to arrange your own sickness cover? The North Korean army maybe? I wonder what level of illness would stop it from being my responsibility. Broken pelvis? Lymphoma? Or just when I was intubated on ITU and denied the power of speech?

Luckily, I could manage to force out a few words in between bouts of vomiting (if not in between bouts of diarrhoea), so I was able to organize a stand-in. I didn't explain what I was doing during the call – it probably sounded like I'd gone paintballing. And I now owe her a shift in return, so it's not even sick *leave*.

I'd always suspected if I ended up off sick it would be work that caused it. My money would have been on some form of emotional collapse, maybe renal failure from dehydration, getting beaten up by an angry relative or smashing my car into a tree after a sleep-deprived night shift. As it happens, it was an altogether stealthier assassin – a portion of noxious homemade moussaka from a labouring patient's mother. I can be fairly sure that was the culprit: it was the only thing I'd managed to eat all day. There should be a saying about Greeks bearing gifts, I thought, shitting through the eye of a hypodermic needle, the taste of bile and faint tinge of aubergine in my throat.

Saturday, 30 September 2006

Review a woman in triage, who just arrived huffing and puffing away in labour. I ask how frequently the contractions are coming and the husband tells me they're three to four times every ten minutes, lasting up to a minute each. I explain I'll need to do an internal examination to assess how far dilated* she is.

The husband tells me he checked before they left home and she was 6 cm. Most dads-to-be don't peek under the hood so I ask him if he's a medic. No, he tells me, he's a plasterer, but 'I know what a centimetre

---

* The contractions of the womb make its neck, or cervix, go from closed before labour to full (10 cm) dilatation at the end of labour, at which point baby can make its grand entrance. The first few centimetres can take an extremely long time, so women aren't generally admitted to labour ward until they're at least 3 cm dilated – like a strange nightclub you can't get into until you've had two gloved fingers in your vagina. Actually, there's probably one of those in Soho already.

is, mate'. I examine the patient and agree with his findings, making him more competent than most of my colleagues.

Saturday, 7 October 2006

I've now spent six months being Simon's on-call mental health helpline since that first Facebook post – any time he's having worrying thoughts, I've told him he can ring me, and he does. I've also told him repeatedly to engage more formally with mental health services, but he's not so keen on listening to that bit. Aside from the fact it's a bit overwhelming to now have a second bleep threatening to go off with bad news any minute, I suspect he can get better help from someone who didn't have to panic-google 'What to say to someone who's suicidal?' But it seems I'm better than nothing – at the very least, he's still alive.

The most stressful part is discovering I've missed a call from him – if I call back too late and he's done himself in, does that make it my fault, like I'm the one who kicked away the chair? I suppose it doesn't, but that's how you feel as a doctor, and probably why I'm in this situation to begin with. If you're the first to notice someone else's patient is breathing strangely or has abnormal blood tests, it's your responsibility to deal with it, or at least ensure someone else does. I'm pretty sure heating engineers don't feel the same way about every kaput boiler they encounter. The difference is obviously the whole 'life and death' thing, which is what separates this job from all others, and makes it so unfathomable to people on the outside.

I call Simon back after a caesarean this evening. I've got my counselling sessions down to about twenty minutes – it's just a case of listening, being sympathetic and reassuring him the feelings will pass. He must realize we have the same chat every time, but it clearly doesn't matter – he just wants to know there's someone out there who cares. And actually, that's a very large part of what being a doctor is.

Monday, 9 October 2006

Today crossed the line from everyday patient idiocy to me checking around the room for hidden cameras. After a lengthy discussion with a patient's husband about how absolutely no condoms fit him, I establish he's pulling them right down over his balls.

Tuesday, 10 October 2006

I missed what the argument was about, but a woman storms out of gynae outpatients screaming at the clinic sister, 'I pay your salary! I pay your salary!' The sister yells back, 'Can I have a raise then?'

Thursday, 19 October 2006

My poker face has served me well over the years. It's seen me through an eighty-year-old telling me about his use of a colossal butt-plug called The Assmaster and gently explaining to a couple in infertility clinic that massaging semen into her navel isn't quite going to cut it, conception-wise. I sit there nodding along blankly like the dog from the Churchill advert. 'And which size of Assmaster, sir?'

Today, however, my poker face cracked. On this morning's ward round, a medical student presented Mrs Ringford – a seventy-year-old gynae patient, recovering on the ward after a posterior repair for a large prolapse.* Unfortunately, he called her 'Mrs Ringpiece' and, much like the patient, I unexpectedly lost my shit.

Monday, 23 October 2006

Called to A&E to review a gentleman in his seventies. I check with the A&E officer that he realizes he's bleeped gynaecology: reviewing a man would be rather pushing my remit. It's complicated, apparently; he'll explain when I get down there.

---

* When you reach a certain age, your body attempts to turn itself inside out via your vagina, but you can avoid all this by performing pelvic floor exercises. There are leaflets that describe these exercises in confusing detail, but I always just used to tell patients, 'Imagine you're sitting in a bath full of eels and you don't want any of them getting in.'

I meet patient NS, a Sikh gentleman who speaks no English at all. He is on holiday, visiting family, and has been unhelpfully accompanied to the hospital by a relative who also speaks no English. His history is therefore taken with the assistance of a telephone interpreter service – in this instance, a Punjabi translator is on the line and the phone is passed back and forth. This particular interpreter may have rather fudged his CV – he seems to be able to speak only slightly more Punjabi than someone who can't speak any Punjabi whatsoever.

The stoic A&E staff have been making glacial progress using the interpreter, and relay what they've established: the patient is bleeding from 'down below', has been doing so for the past week and – crucially to my attendance – is a hermaphrodite.* I tell the A&E officer that I sincerely doubt this elderly bearded man is part of the intersex community, and ask to speak to the interpreter.

'Can you ask if the patient has a womb?' The phone gets passed back, and the patient starts to repeat a word to us very loudly and angrily in Punjabi. The patient furiously unbuttons his shirt to reveal a Port-a-Cath† –

---

* Hermaphroditism is a very rare intersex disorder where the patient possesses both testicular and ovarian tissue. It's named after the Greek legend of Hermaphroditus, who was said to be both male and female. He/she was the son/daughter of Hermes and Aphrodite, who it must be said had a pretty lazy system for naming their children.

† A Port-a-Cath is a device that sits under the skin to allow easy

our eureka moment. In unison we all say, 'Haemophiliac!' and I leave them to deal with his rectal bleed.

Tuesday, 31 October 2006

Moral maze. In the labour ward dressing rooms after a long shift. I'm leaving at 10 p.m. rather than 8 p.m. thanks to a major obstetric haemorrhage ending up back in theatre. I'm meant to be going to a Halloween party, but now I don't have time to go home and pick up my costume. However, I am currently dressed in scrubs and splattered head to toe in blood. Would it be *so* wrong?

Saturday, 4 November 2006

Get bleeped to see a postnatal patient at 1 a.m. The ODP* relays to the bleeping midwife that I'm in the middle of a caesarean. I get bleeped again at 1.15 a.m. (still doing the section) and 1.30 a.m. (writing up my operation notes). Eventually, I head off to review the patient. The big emergency? She's going home in the morning and wants to have her passport application countersigned by a doctor while she's still in here.

---

injection of drugs and taking of blood, for people who need it done frequently.

* An Operating Department Practitioner (ODP) is Muttley to the anaesthetist's Dick Dastardly.

Wednesday, 15 November 2006

I have entered the MRCOG* Part One exam. A textbook advises me to try a past paper before I start revising – 'You might be pleasantly surprised how much you already know!' I attempt one.

March 1997, Paper 1, Question 1.

True or false? Chromaffin cells:

A. Are innervated by pre-ganglionic sympathetic nerve fibres

B. Are present in the adrenal cortex

C. Are derived from neuro-ectoderm

D. Can decarboxylate amino acids

E. Are present in coeliac ganglia

Aside from the fact I know what less than half of these words mean (and most of those are prepositions), I can't help wondering how it's relevant to my baby-delivering abilities. But if it's what my insane demonic overlords want me to know, who am I to argue?

Another textbook cheerily informs me that 'It's quite possible to revise for MRCOG Part One in just six months, with an hour or two's study every evening.' It's

---

* Member of the Royal College of Obstetricians and Gynaecologists – a necessary hurdle to proceed up the ranks. The exam is in two equally brutal parts, and feels rather like the Labours of Hercules, in that you're forced to do it to demonstrate your extraordinary dedication to the field more than anything else.

one of those phrases that is intended to be reassuring but has the opposite effect, like 'it's only a small tumour' or 'most of the fire's been put out already'.

I'm not entirely sure where these extra couple of hours a day are going to come from – either I need to give up my frivolous hobby of sleeping or cut out my commute by living in a store cupboard at work. Oh, and my exam's in four months, not six.

Monday, 25 December 2006

I don't particularly mind working Christmas Day – there are snacks everywhere, people on the whole are in a good mood and there are very few worried well.[*] Generally nobody rocks up as a patient on Christmas Day unless they're genuinely sick, genuinely in labour or genuinely hate their family. (In which case, we've at least got some common ground.) I'm not convinced H sees it this way, as we exchange gifts at breakneck speed before 7 a.m.

Tradition at St Agatha's dictates that the on-call consultant[†] turns up and does a ward round on Christmas

---

[*] A lot of individuals (I'm not calling them patients; there's nothing wrong with them) come to hospital under the misapprehension they're in any way ill – known as the worried well. If this is because of something they've read online, they're called cyberchondriacs.

[†] Consultants are generally on call from home outside of normal working hours, giving telephone advice when needed, and only coming in for major emergencies.

Day, which eases the workload for the juniors. The consultant will also bring a bag of presents for the patients – toiletries, panettone, that sort of thing – because, well, it's pretty rotten being a hospital inpatient over Christmas, and the little things do make a difference. Best of all, tradition has it that this consultant will be dressed as Santa Claus as they do their round.

The nursing staff's disappointment is palpable when today's consultant, Mr Hopkirk, turns up around 10 a.m. wearing chinos and a jumper. Before the cries of 'Grinch!' and 'Ebeneezer!' get too deafening, he explains that the last time he was on call on Christmas Day, he chucked on the outfit and beard for the ward round and was halfway through when an elderly patient suddenly went into cardiac arrest, so he dashed over and started CPR while a nurse went to fetch the trolley. Unusually, the CPR was successful,* and the patient gasped back to life to the sight of a six-foot Santa liplocked with her, his arms on her chest. 'I can still hear her scream,' he said.

---

* If your heart stops, you're probably going to die. God is fairly strict on that matter. If you collapse on the street and a bystander starts CPR then your chance of survival is around 8 per cent. In hospital, with trained personnel, drugs and defibrillators, it's only about twice that. People don't realize quite how horrific resuscitation is – undignified, brutal and with a fairly woeful success rate. When discussing Do Not Resuscitate orders, relatives often want 'everything to be done' without really knowing what that means. Really, the form should say, 'If your mother's heart stops, would you like us to break all her ribs and electrocute her?'

'Go on,' says one of the nurses, like a child failing to hide their distress that their Christmas present is a calligraphy set not a kitten. 'Maybe just the hat?'

Wednesday, 17 January 2007

'In order to encourage use of public transport' there is no staff car park at the hospital – an admirable sentiment that would land me with a two-hour-twenty-minute commute each way. Instead, I've opted for a seventy-minute drive, leaving my wheels in the visitors' car park. The pricing system must have been dreamt up by someone who realized their chances of winning the lottery more than once were pretty skeletal, and thought there must be another way to raise a similar annual revenue. It's £3 per hour, with no discount for long stays, and is applicable every hour of every day and every night, except for Christmas, which presumably they decided would be greedy.

The only exception is for women in labour, who get a parking voucher valid for three days when signed by the labour ward supervisor. I'm on good terms with the supervisors – not so much for the fact that day in, day out I resolve obstetric emergencies, but because I occasionally bring in a box of Viennese whirls. As a result they're happy to sign me a parking voucher every few days, and have therefore provided me with a *marché-gris* parking space for the past few months.

Today, however, the jig is up: my car has a clamp and

a £120 fine for removal jammed under the windscreen wiper. I weigh up buying an angle-grinder for fifty quid, but I've been at work twelve hours and just want to get to bed as quickly as possible. I grab the notice to find out who to call. The parking attendant has scrawled on the back, 'Long fucking labour, pal.'

Sunday, 21 January 2007

Just when I was thinking it had been a while since the last episode of 'unexpected objects stuck in orifices', today a patient in her twenties presents to A&E unable to retrieve a bottle she'd put up there. Speculum* in – so what's it going to be this time? Chanel No. 5? Two litres of Tizer? The magic potion I need to drink to take me to the next level of that Dungeons & Dragons game I abandoned twenty-four years ago? As it transpires, it's a medical sample bottle, filled to the top with urine.

I can't work out the backstory, so ask her to enlighten me. It turns out she has to provide her probation officer with clean urine samples, and so, rather than choose the simpler option of not taking drugs, she has her mother piss in a pot for her, which she then smuggles in vagi-

---

* The speculum is a great clanking duckbill of a device used for looking inside the vagina. The first speculum was invented by an American surgeon called Sims back in 1845. He later wrote in his autobiography, 'If there was anything I hated, it was investigating the organs of the female pelvis', which goes some way to explain why he devised such a hideous instrument.

nally and decants into the sample pot she gets given by the probation officer. I think about the enormous volume of paperwork I'll generate for myself if I document this in the notes, so pretend I never asked the question and send her home.

Monday, 29 January 2007

My favourite patient died a couple of weeks ago, and it rather knocked the stuffing out of me. It was far from unexpected: KL was eighty in the shade, with metastatic ovarian cancer, and she'd been on the ward as long as I've worked on this unit, minus a couple of short-lived discharges home. Five foot nothing of Polish sass, with bright, twinkling eyes, she loved to tell long, meandering stories from back home that she would invariably lose interest in the moment they got interesting – almost all of them ended with 'blah blah blah' and a vague wave of the hand.

Best of all, she despised my consultant, Prof. Fletcher. She called him 'old man' every time she saw him even though she had a good fifteen years on him, regularly prodded her finger into his chest when making a point, and once asked to see his line manager. I'd genuinely look forward to her stop on the ward round – we'd always have a good natter and I really felt like I'd got to know her.

She immediately clocked I was Polish, despite three generations of my family living in England, breeding with Brits and sending their offspring to expensive schools. She asks my original family name – I tell her it's Strykowski. She thinks it's sad a good Polish name like that is out of commission; I should be proud of my heritage and change it back.[*]

Over the months I'd met all of her children, as well as numerous friends and neighbours who came to visit. '*Now* they like me!' she would say. Despite the joke, you could see why everyone did; she had a magnetic personality.

I was really upset when I heard she'd died. I decided I should go to the funeral – it felt like the right thing to do. I swapped out of clinic this afternoon so I could make it, and let Prof. Fletcher know I'd be attending, as a courtesy.

He told me I couldn't – doctors don't go to their patients' funerals, it's unprofessional. I didn't quite understand why. His argument hinged on drawing a personal and professional line, which I agree with to an extent, but his tone seemed to suggest I was going along in order to seduce her grandchildren or get myself written into the will. I suspect that underpinning it is actually an old-fashioned sense that doctors have 'lost' or 'failed' if a patient dies; there's an element of blame or shame. Not really a sustainable attitude in gynae oncology, where there's always going to be quite a high patient

---

[*] Strykowski is pronounced Strike-Offski, so I'm not convinced it's a great name for a doctor.

turnover. I was disappointed – partly because I'd had a suit dry-cleaned specially – but he's my boss and those were his very clear instructions.

Of course, I went to the funeral all the same – not least because that's exactly the kind of 'fuck you' she'd have wanted to give him. It was a beautiful service, and I'm certain it was the right thing to do – for me, and for the friends and family I'd met on the ward. Plus I was able to sleep with one of her grandchildren.*

---

* 'I think you should point out that this is a joke,' recommended one of the lawyers.

4

Senior House Officer – Post Three

I realize everyone moans about their salary and thinks they deserve more, but I'm happy to look back on my time as an SHO with a bit of objectivity and declare I was profoundly underpaid. The money is utterly out of step with the level of responsibility you have – literally life and death decisions – plus there's the fact you've been to medical school for six years, worked as a doctor for three and started to accrue postgraduate qualifications. Even if you think it's appropriate that you take home less money per week than a train driver, there's still the fact that these working weeks can involve over a hundred hours of unremitting slog, meaning the parking meters outside the hospital are on a better hourly rate.

Doctors tend not to complain about the money though. It's not a profession you go into to satisfy the dollar signs behind your eyes, whatever the occasional dead-mouthed politician may say. Besides, even if you're unhappy with your salary, there's sod all you can do about it. It's all determined centrally, and rolled out across the entire profession. Perhaps it's unhelpful to describe it as a salary – the NHS should call what they pay doctors a 'stipend', acknowledge it's below the prevailing rate but that they're in the job because it's their calling, rather than for any financial imperative.[*]

Nothing about the job plays along with the conventional reward structure for employees. There's no opportunity for a bonus – the closest that exists is 'ash cash', where juniors get £40 a pop for signing a form for the funeral directors to confirm the patient about to be cremated doesn't have a pacemaker fitted. (Pacemakers explode during the process, taking with them entire crematoria and congregations, as one family presumably found out during a particularly stressful funeral.) Thinking about it, that's pretty much the opposite of performance-related pay. There's no dazzling your superiors and leapfrogging your peers, or any opportunity for promotion: you progress up the ranks at a regulation rate.

Everyone seems to think doctors get upgraded on planes, but the only way that happens in reality is if they put on a suit – and then apply for a job in the City, earn more money and buy a business-class ticket. I suppose you do have unlimited access to the informal medical opinions of every speciality at work if you begin to malfunction in any way. This is good, but just as well, as there's little chance you'd get the time off work to go

---

[*] Like the way priests get a stipend for their duty to God (or love of choir boys, depending on denomination).

to an outpatient clinic. But I'm not sure it's worth the flip side of providing medical advice to every friend at every opportunity. You'll hear 'Could you just take a quick look?' more than you'll ever hear 'Hey, it's great to see you.'* My only small consolation was not having to give medical advice to relatives, what with most of my relatives being doctors.

All medics get to grips with the lack of promotion and financial incentives, but it's harder to accept the fact that it's rare to get a 'well done'. The butlers at Buckingham Palace, under orders to float out of rooms backwards and never to make eye contact with the Queen, probably get more recognition. It didn't strike me for years, until the fifth or sixth time I'd had my knuckles rapped for some trivial fuck-up when a degree of human error had kicked in, that none of my consultants had ever taken me aside to say I was doing a good job. Or that I'd made a smart management decision, saved a life, cleverly thought on my feet or stayed at work late for the thirtieth consecutive shift without complaining. Nobody joins the NHS looking for plaudits or expecting a gold star or a biscuit every time they do a good job, but you'd think it might be basic psychology (and common sense) to occasionally acknowledge, if not reward, good behaviour to get the most out of your staff.

---

* Tediously, this has morphed into something even worse now I'm a TV writer. I'd take 'What do you think about this rash?' over 'What do you think about this script?' any day.

Patients tended to get it, though. When one of them said thank you, you knew they meant it – even if it felt like it wasn't for anything special, just one of the smaller horrors thrown at you that day. I've kept every single card a patient has given me. Birthday and Christmas cards from family and friends would always get thrown away, but these guys survived every house move, escaping even my cathartic clear-out of medical paperwork once it was all over. They were little fist-bumps that kept me going, rays of thoughtfulness from my patients that hit the spot when bosses couldn't, or wouldn't, oblige.

It took until now, my third job as an SHO, to feel properly recognized by a consultant for the first time. A few months through my contract, my clinical supervisor said that a registrar was leaving the post early for a research job, and asked if I'd be interested in acting up on the rota. She told me she'd been very impressed with my work in the department. I knew this was a lie; she'd met me twice – once at induction and once to bollock me for starting a patient on oral rather than intravenous antibiotics. She'd clearly just looked through everyone's CVs and clocked that I had worked as an SHO for the longest. But sometimes it doesn't matter how they spot you as long as they actually *do*, so I beamed and said I'd be delighted.

I also realized this could make a significant practical difference to me. Three years into our relationship, H and I were taking the next step into adulthood and looking to buy a flat. I'd decided to sacrifice a shorter commute so we could have a permanent base, a place to actually call home, somewhere you can hang a picture on the wall without being docked fifty quid from your rental deposit. Most non-medical friends were clambering onto the second rung of the property ladder by then, and you know what it's like when your friends are all doing something and you're not. Whether it's fingering someone at a party, taking your driving test or dropping hundreds of thousands of pounds on a dungeon with dry rot – nobody wants to be left behind.

Because every penny of salary helps with getting a mortgage, I asked the consultant if I'd be paid on the registrar scale while I was acting up. She laughed so long and so hard I'm pretty sure you could hear it through two sets of double doors over on labour ward.

Monday, 12 February 2007

Prescribing a morning-after pill in A&E. The patient says, 'I slept with three guys last night. Will one pill be enough?'

Thursday, 22 February 2007

Spent the morning going through three months of bank statements with the mortgage broker so he can assess my expenditure. 'You don't . . . go out much, do you?' he says, totting it up. For once I'm grateful for my job – we wouldn't have saved up enough for a deposit if I was allowed the normal social life of someone in their late twenties.

It's reasonably depressing looking at where the money goes: a lot of coffee, a lot of petrol, a lot of take-away pizza – necessities and practicalities. Not much in the way of fun or extracurricular frippery – no pubs, restaurants, cinemas or holidays. Hang on, what's that? There we go – theatre tickets! Shortly followed by a payment to a florist, after bailing on H at the last minute. Depressingly, it happens frequently enough that I can't even remember the particular emergency or staffing crisis on that occasion.

Wednesday, 28 February 2007

In gynae clinic, I go online to look up some management guidelines for a patient. The trust's IT department
has blocked the Royal College of Obstetrics and Gynaecology website and classified it as 'pornography'.

Monday, 12 March 2007

Pretty sure that if obs and gynae goes arse over tit I
could retrain in psychiatry in about fifteen minutes –
I've basically taught myself how to do it over the course
of a dozen conversations with Simon. Tonight I was
pretty stressed when he called and had a bit of a moan
about work. Unexpectedly, this really seemed to help
him. Either he's a horrible sadist and likes the idea of me
having an awful day or it's comforting for him to know
that everyone else has shit going on in their lives too.
Misery loves company, after all – you only have to look
in the doctors' mess to know that.

Maybe it's like when you're in a proper relationship
for the first time and you meet their family – and you
see it's not just *your* family that's a miserable fucked-up
mess with dozens of dark secrets and grotesque dinner-
table habits. We finished today's call with Simon in
hysterics after I told him a lump of placenta flew into
my mouth during a manual removal and I had to go to
occupational health about it. He may well be a sadist,
come to think of it.

Thursday, 15 March 2007

I ask a patient in antenatal clinic how many weeks she is now. There's a long pause. Cogs turn. A camera slowly pans across a wasteland. Maths isn't everyone's strong point, but I'm after the number between six and forty that people must constantly ask her about. Finally:

'In total?'

Yes, in total.

'God, I couldn't even tell you in months . . .'

Has she got amnesia? Is she a clone of another woman currently being held prisoner in an evil sci-fi villain's lair? I start to ask when her last period was, and she interrupts.

'Well, I'm thirty-two in June, so that's got to be more than a thousand weeks . . .'

Christ.

Thursday, 22 March 2007

Idea for *Dragons' Den*: a bleep with a snooze button.

Thursday, 5 April 2007

Revenge is a dish best served cold – so long as it doesn't end up poisoning the wrong person. I was called to review a patient on the ward: she'd had a laparoscopic drainage of a pelvic abscess in the morning and her pulse had been raised all evening. Looking through her notes, this lady was in her mid-fifties and had discovered on her wedding anniversary that she wasn't the only person to have received a pearl necklace from her husband. Her reaction was seemingly straight out of niche porn – she took herself, and her husband's credit card, off to Trinidad and Tobago and had sex with as many men as she could over the course of a fortnight, expanding her bedroom (and beach) repertoire to include anal sex.

Back home, bow-legged but unbowed, she soon found she was having terrible abdominal pain, plus producing purulent monsoons from both her Trinidad *and* her Tobago. She was diagnosed with pelvic inflammatory disease,* and even IV antibiotics couldn't persuade it to sod off – seemingly there's some pretty weapons-grade gonorrhoea going round the Caribbean. Today's procedure would hopefully get her back on the road.

It turned out her raised pulse wasn't caused by any surgical complications, but because she was in floods of tears. I asked what was up and she told me her eighteen-year-old son was coming over tomorrow to visit, and she didn't know what to say to him – how would he react when he found out why she was in hospital? I

---

* Pelvic inflammatory disease, or PID, is when untreated gonorrhoea or chlamydia spreads north and gunks up the pelvic organs – it can be tricky to treat and even result in permanent pelvic pain. It's also one of the main causes of female infertility. Basically, use condoms, or you might end up not needing them at all.

reassured her that an eighteen-year-old boy would rather peel his testicles and douse them in malt vinegar than ask any questions at all about why his mother is on a gynaecology ward. The phrase 'women's problems' alone – especially if delivered in hushed tones while staring straight into his eyes – will have him changing the subject immediately, even if he has to start a small fire as a distraction. Tears over and pulse back down to normal. Although she might want to think up a plausible excuse for that incredible suntan . . .

Monday, 9 April 2007

Results out today. I have somehow passed my MRCOG Part One exam and am celebrating in the pub with Ron. Unfortunately, drinks are strictly non-alcoholic as I have to head straight off afterwards to a night shift, and I gather turning up drunk is frowned upon. Ron recently got through his postgraduate accountancy exams, so we compare notes. While his firm cut down his hours so he could revise, I had to squeeze in as much revision as my bloodshot eyes would allow after work. Ron had a full month of study leave before the exam; I applied for a week off, but rota gaps meant that it ended up getting cancelled at the last minute, without discussion. His firm paid for all exam fees and materials; I had to shell out for £300-worth of textbooks, a £500 course, £100 for online learning resources and £400 on the exam itself, a grand total of £1,300 – a mere two-thirds of my monthly take-home pay.

My carefully considered answers don't even get seen by a human – it's a multiple-choice paper and you fill in the answers in pencil on a grid, which then gets scanned and marked by a computer. I show Ron the RCOG pencil I pinched.

He immediately gets a promotion and pay rise for passing his exam; all mine means is that I'm now eligible to enter the Part Two exam.

'No. All it means,' says Ron sympathetically, 'is that you spent £1,300 on a pencil.'

Thursday, 19 April 2007

An email from Infection Control informs all doctors that long-sleeved shirts are now banned in clinical environments. Some study has swabbed a bunch of cuffs and discovered it would be more hygienic for us to wear shirts made out of fresh human faeces and poorly sealed vials of ebola. The same apparently applies to neckties, which dangle down, bobbing in and out of various festering wounds and cross-pollinating bugs across the hospital like polyester honeybees with a death wish.

We are henceforth instructed to wear short-sleeved shirts, so I brush aside any hope of making the cover of *Vogue* while at work and go shopping to invest my savings in five of the things. These short-sleeved numbers, we are told, may be worn either with no tie or with a bow tie – giving us the option of dressing like an airline steward or a paedophile. I'll go without, thanks. Tea? Coffee? Hot towel?

Wednesday, 2 May 2007

I finish consenting a couple for caesarean section. 'Any questions at all?' I ask the room.

'Yes,' chips in their six-year-old. 'Do you think Jesus was black?'

Saturday, 5 May 2007

In lieu of an incentive scheme at work, I've invented my own perks: I take scrubs home for pyjamas and steal the odd patient meal at night. It's 1 a.m., I'm absolutely starving and it's my only chance for some food for the next seven hours, so I sidle into the gynae ward kitchen. Clearly I'm not the only one with an eye for a freebie – there's a new sign up on the fridge warning staff that meals are strictly for patients only. As security systems go it's not exactly sophisticated – they may struggle to prevent the more determined thief with A4 paper, Blu Tack and Comic Sans alone.

Tonight's delicacy is 'Quorn-style Savoury Mince with Sultanas'. It's like they got Accenture in to come up with the least appealing possible menu options. I think I'll just take my chances and let nervous energy and Red Bull keep me going.

Saturday, 12 May 2007

My philosophy on flights is to get so hammered that no right-minded air steward would want me anywhere near a sick passenger, which has served me well these past few years.* Karma repaid me tonight, not on the flight itself but twelve hours later, in Glasgow for the weekend and walking back to the hotel after dinner and drinks and drinks and drinkssssss with Ron and his wife Hannah.

Walking down Bath Street at 1 a.m., we see three guys in their late teens hanging around some basement steps, outside a shop door, surrounded by an extraordinary amount of blood. It looked unreal, like a murder scene on a Channel 5 drama. They were all the worse for wear – though probably no worse than any of us – and one was exsanguinating from what looked like a big arterial bleed on his forearm. Impossible to guess how much blood was sprayed and pooled around, but it couldn't have been less than a litre. He was conscious, though barely, and nothing was being done to stem the blood loss.

---

* My family are much nicer people than me. One Christmas, British Airways sent my dad a pair of return tickets to anywhere in the world as a thank you for answering the 'Is there a doctor on board?' call, and handing out some antihistamines from the medicine box. My brother (also a GP) was extremely unimpressed – he'd spent the entire duration of a budget airline flight managing an urgent cardiac situation with extremely limited resources and didn't even get the words 'thank you' as a thank you, let alone a free trip to Bali.

I sobered up extremely quickly and told them I was a doctor. The friends were pointing at the smashed glass door and repeatedly telling me he'd tripped and fallen, as if the fact he'd clearly broken into a newsagent was anyone's main concern here. They'd called an ambulance already, but I had Ron phone 999 to expedite its appearance and asked Hannah to rip up T-shirts to make tourniquets. I held the guy's arm up high and squeezed hard. His pulse was slow and thready,* and he was drifting in and out of consciousness. I keep talking, talking, talking – telling him the ambulance is really close, I'm a doctor, everything's going to be fine. It doesn't matter how many times you say it or whether any of it is true – well, at least the 'doctor' part is true – you have to believe it, because *they* need to believe it.

It felt like he was on the brink of cardiac arrest and I was going through CPR in my head so I didn't need to think twice when he did. Was this even legal – drunk in charge of an emergency? I was confident I was managing the situation correctly, but it wouldn't look *great* if he died with me in this state. Mercifully, the ambulance arrived almost immediately and they whisked him away, filling him with the fluids he needed to save his life. All's well that ends well, but I had a terrible feeling of

---

* If you lose blood, then your pulse usually speeds up – your heart needs to work extra hard to get oxygen around the body given there's less blood to transport it. When the pulse becomes slow in this situation, it generally means the body is getting exhausted and preparing to throw in the towel.

impotence waiting for the ambulance to pull up. Back in the hotel I poured myself a £12 miniature from the minibar and realized that even on a plane I'd have had more resources to help him. The whisky would have been cheaper, too.

Monday, 14 May 2007

In the doctors' mess, my friend Zac – currently working in orthopaedics – tells me that he always muddles the words 'shoulder' and 'elbow' in his mind, and has to really concentrate before using either term. Before I even have time to process this and what it could mean for his next patient, an intensive care registrar joins in from the next sofa: since childhood, she's always malapropped the words 'coma' and 'cocoon'. The more she tries to remember which is which, the more her mind convinces her she's got it the wrong way round. She shows us a piece of paper in her wallet that reads,

COCOON = Insect
COMA = Patient.

This, we hear, helps prevent the admittedly hilarious scenario of sitting down an inconsolable relative to break the news that their husband is in a cocoon.

Tuesday, 12 June 2007

It's five minutes until my shift ends and I need to get away on time to go out for dinner. Naturally, I'm asked to review a patient – she's got a second-degree tear,[*] and the midwife looking after her tells me she hasn't been signed off to repair those yet.[†]

Me: 'I haven't been signed off to do them either.'

Midwife: 'You don't need to get signed off to do things – you're a doctor.' (Depressing but true.)

Me: 'Isn't there another midwife who can do it?'

Midwife: 'She's on her break.'

Me: 'I'm on my break.' (Untrue.)

Midwife: 'You don't get breaks.' (Depressing but true.)

Me: (pleading, in a tone of voice I've never managed before, like I've unlocked a secret level of my vocal cords) 'But it's my *birthday*.' (Depressing but true.)

Midwife: 'It's labour ward – it's always someone's birthday.'

---

[*] Having a baby can rip your undercarriage to shreds, there's no getting away from it, especially if you're a first-time mum. Durex should take their cue from cigarette manufacturers and show photos of post-partum perineums on their packaging – no woman could look at that and ever risk getting pregnant. A first-degree tear goes through the skin, a second-degree tear goes into the perineal muscles, a third-degree tear involves the anal sphincter and a fourth-degree tear rips your leg off or something.

[†] Doctors' and midwives' roles are fairly well defined in most aspects of labour ward – midwives are responsible for normal deliveries; doctors are involved when there are worries about mum or baby's well-being or the progress of labour. Who gets the sewing kit out for first- and second-degree tears is a greyer area than your nan's vagina.

Tuesday, 19 June 2007

An email to all clinical staff, letting us know a psychiatric inpatient has been transferred to the respiratory ward following a diagnosis of pneumonia. But this wasn't the kind of 'say hello if you see him' notice you'd get if a new kid transferred to your school. Yesterday it was discovered he'd been wandering around the ward minesweeping like the last aunt at a wedding, downing the contents of every sputum pot he found on fellow patients' bedside tables.

We are advised to send all clinical samples *immediately* to the lab and not to leave any in easy reach for the time being. Someone has replied-all with 'Yuck', which feels rather like watching a nuclear reactor explode and saying 'Oh dear'.

Tuesday, 26 June 2007

I've been in the doghouse for days now. We were at H's friend Luna's house – Luna is pregnant, and just before dinner she whipped out a photo album of their recent 3-D scans. I suspected my thoughts on 3-D scans – that they serve no purpose other than keeping 3-D scanning companies rich, and boring the anuses off dinner-party guests – would go down like a cup of cold sick, so I had a polite flick through along with everyone else.

'Everything seem OK?' Luna asked me. I wanted to say, 'Looks the same as they all fucking do,' but I suspected that might lose the room, so I just smiled sweetly, handed the photos back and said, 'She looks perfect.' The temperature in the room dropped about ten degrees and murder flashed discernibly across Luna's eyes. 'She? SHE?'

It's the first time I've dropped the ball on this, so to speak, and worst of all with a friend, not a patient. Dinner felt like it took a fortnight; eye contact avoided, plates plomped unceremoniously in front of me.

It didn't help that tensions were already running high at home. Two weeks ago, our flat purchase fell through. It seems that, with a total disregard for my blood pressure and a relationship slightly fraying at the edges, the owners have decided not to sell it after all. I rather suspect they've merely decided not to sell it to *us*, probably because someone else had offered them a bit more money. Luckily, we've only spent a couple of thousand fucking pounds on solicitors and surveys and whatnot. I know more about this flat – that I will now never set foot in again – than I do about any of my closest blood relations. Everyone tells us that these things happen for a reason. In our case, the reason is that the world favours bastards and clearly wants us to spend our every spare moment with estate agents for the next few months.

But life goes on, even if it's peppered with annoying reminders. The depleted bank account, for one, and the fact that, unless I take a five-minute PTSD-avoiding detour, I drive past the flat that got away every morning on my journey to work. And today – amazingly, just to prove there's no escape – the couple who screwed us over turned up in antenatal clinic. I'd not met them before, but here was their address in front of me, the exact same address that's permanently scarring my happiness.

In a Tarantino movie, this would be the part where I produce two samurai swords and unleash a ten-minute tirade about honour, vengeance and respect, before decapitating them. In reality I just said, 'Hi, I'm Adam – one of the doctors,' and they had no idea. Issues of morality, probity and legality sadly restrict revenge opportunities to near enough zero, so I conducted their appointment to the best of my abilities, albeit through gritted teeth. I wasn't 100 per cent sure that the baby was cephalic,* so I quickly ran the scanner over the mother. Baby was the right way up and all was well. 'Do you want to see the heart beating?' I asked them. 'There it is – all looks normal there. There's an arm, another arm, that's a leg, that's his penis . . . Oh, didn't you know?'

---

* Cephalic means baby is head down – this is normal. The opposite is breech, meaning bum first. Breech presentation occurs in 3 per cent of pregnancies, and famous examples include Emperor Nero, Kaiser Wilhelm, Frank Sinatra and Billy Joel. If you win a pub quiz off the back of this, you owe me a pint.

Saturday, 30 June 2007

A news story in the paper about a hospital porter who's been jailed for pretending to be a doctor for the last few years. Just finished one of those shifts where I wondered if I could get away with pretending to be a porter.

Tuesday, 10 July 2007

I clearly need to change my patter. It usually goes something like: 'I couldn't see anything on the ultrasound just by looking with a probe on the tummy – doesn't mean there's anything to worry about, early pregnancies can often be very difficult to see this way. Would it be OK if I did an ultrasound using an internal probe to get a better view?'

After today's incident, should my licence to practise remain intact, my new spiel will be: 'I couldn't see anything on the ultrasound just by looking with a probe on the tummy – doesn't mean there's anything to worry about, early pregnancies can often be very difficult to see this way. Would it be OK if I did an ultrasound using an internal probe to get a better view? In a few seconds' time I'm going to rummage in a drawer and pull out a condom and a sachet of KY jelly. Just to be clear: the condom is a cover for the ultrasound probe and the KY jelly is to lubricate it. When you see what's in my hands, please do not scream so loudly that three members of staff come rushing into the room.'

Monday, 23 July 2007

Sending a patient home from the day surgery unit following laparoscopic sterilization. I tell her she can have sex again as soon as she feels ready, but to use alternative contraception until her next period. I nod at her husband and say, 'That means *he* has to wear a condom.' I can't quite work out why their faces are a picture of horror, melting like the Nazis at the end of *Raiders of the Lost Ark*. What have I said? It's perfectly good advice, right? I look at them both again, and realize the man is actually her father.

Tuesday, 31 July 2007

One of the house officers turned up in A&E last night, having attempted suicide with an overdose of anti-depressants. There's a shared sense of numbness amongst the doctors. The only surprise is it doesn't happen more often – you're given huge responsibility, minimal supervision and absolutely no pastoral support.* You work yourself to exhaustion, pushing yourself beyond what could be reasonably expected of you, and end up constantly feeling like you don't know what you're doing.

---

* A 2015 study by the Medical Protection Society showed that 85 per cent of doctors have experienced mental health issues, and 13 per cent admitted to suicidal feelings. A 2009 paper in the *British Journal of Psychiatry* showed that young female doctors in the UK are two and a half times more likely than other women to kill themselves.

Sometimes it just feels that way, and you're actually doing fine – and sometimes you *really* don't know what you're doing.

Happily, this occasion is the latter, and she has taken a completely harmless dose of antidepressants. In any other profession, if someone's job drove them to attempt suicide, you'd expect some kind of inquiry into what happened and a concerted effort to make sure it never happened again. Yet nobody said anything – we all just heard from friends, like we were in the school playground. I doubt we'd have got so much as an email if she'd died. I'm pretty unshockable, but I'll never cease to be amazed by hospitals' wilful ineptitude when it comes to caring for their own staff.

5

Registrar – Post One

As a house officer you think your registrar is unim-peachably correct and clever, like God maybe, or Google, and you try not to bother them under almost any circumstance. As an SHO, they're your port of call whenever you get stuck and need an answer: the safety net of some wise words just a quick bleep away. And then, before you know it, the registrar is *you*.

In obs and gynae, it means you'll frequently be the most senior person in clinic. You'll lead the ward rounds more often than not. You get to be called Mr Kay rather than Dr – which makes the previous decade of studying feel like a fucking waste of time. You're expected to teach medical students. You're expected to perform all but the meatiest of operations. Most crucially, you run the labour ward. There are senior registrars and poten-tially even consultants available if you hit DEFCON 1, but this is the grade where you're generally responsible for keeping a dozen labouring mums and babies alive at all times. This one probably needs a caesarean, these two are going to need an instrumental delivery, this one's haemorrhaging. You become amazing at prioritizing. It's like you're living in a constant logic puzzle; the one with the boat, the fox, the chicken and the bag of grain. Except there are a dozen chickens, they're all delivering triplets and the boat's made of sugar.

It sounds horrific – and at times it was – but the day I started as a registrar, I had a huge spring in my step. Not since the day I qualified had I felt so optimistic – I was practically shitting confetti. I was suddenly halfway to becoming a consultant, enjoying the Wednesday afternoon of my metaphorical week. Not only was a senior job just a few years away, I could actually picture myself doing it, maybe even doing it well. It felt like everything at work and home was clicking into place, like I'd finally figured out I'd been holding the map upside down all this time. For once my life didn't seem that depressing compared to non-medic friends. I had a flat, I had a new(er) car and a (more or less) stable relationship. I felt satisfied. Not smug or complacent, but just in marked contrast to the years I'd felt somehow *unsatisfied* with the way things had been going.

I realized that most of my colleagues weren't so lucky, especially when it came to their home lives. Mine was largely held together by superhuman levels of tolerance and understanding; most doctors' relationships crumbled after a year or so – the cracks that they all develop would appear far too early, like some bizarre premature ageing disorder.

Certainly the hours don't help. After four or five years of intravenous NHS Kool-Aid, staying late, arriving early and filling in for colleagues have become fully formed habits. A widely held belief among non-medics is that there's some degree of choice involved in coming home at 10 p.m. rather than 8 p.m. But really the only choice is whether you fuck over yourself or your patients. The former is annoying, the latter means that people die – so it's not really a choice at all. The system runs on skeleton staff and, on all but the quietest shifts, relies on the charity of doctors staying beyond their contracted hours to get things done. It would be against everything you stand for to knowingly compromise patient safety, so you don't – which means you stay late after almost every shift. Of course, medics aren't alone in working late – you could say the same of lawyers and bankers – but at least they can become 'weekend warriors', letting down their hair and their ancestors in a forty-eight-hour blast of unremitting hedonism. Our weekends were usually spent at work.

But it's more than just the hours; you're generally no fun to be around when you get home. You're exhausted, you're snappy from a stressful day and you even manage to deny your partner their normal post-work chat of bitching about their colleagues. They know as soon as they start on their workplace quibbles – which presumably don't involve any near-death experiences, unless they're a tightrope walker, firefighter or counter staff at a drive-thru Burger King – you'll reflexively man that old ship *One-Up* and talk about the horrors of your own day.

Your subconscious ends up making a decision on your behalf. Either you fail to tune out the bad stuff from work and become permanently distracted and haunted at home or you develop a hardened emotional exoskeleton, which apparently isn't considered an ideal quality in a partner.

A few of my colleagues had kids by this point and lived their lives in constant childcare hell, adding 'guilt' to the psychology textbook of emotions that a career in medicine bequeaths you. I don't have kids, but I could understand what a gut-wrench it was for my colleagues to settle for a goodnight phone call with their children rather than tucking them in and reading them *The Gruffalo*. Or, more often than not, they'd miss the call altogether because labour ward was in meltdown. A friend who worked in general surgery once couldn't go along to his own son's emergency surgery because he was performing non-emergency surgery on someone else's son and no one could cover for him.

Once I became a registrar, I noticed the interesting paradox that while you become an expert in prioritizing at work, you generally become even worse at prioritizing in real life. But for a while there I felt like the exception who proved the rule – the one guy who had his shit together in some small way, plates all spinning away nicely. Now I just had to make sure none of them smashed . . .

Thursday, 16 August 2007

A horror story. Patient GL, whose genetic make-up appears to be 50 per cent goji berry recipes and 50 per cent Mumsnet posts, has announced she wants to eat her placenta. The midwife and I both pretend not to hear this – firstly because we don't know what the hospital protocol is, and secondly because it's completely revolting. GL calls it 'placentophagia' to make it sound more official, which doesn't particularly wash; you can make anything sound official by translating it into the ancient Greek.*

She explains how natural it is among other mammals, which is another somewhat defective argument – we don't let other mammals do things like run for parliament or drive buses, nor do we normalize other things they do like fucking the furniture or eating their young (or 'paedophagia', as she'd presumably call it).

I turn the conversation to the more pressing matter of clapping some forceps on her baby's head and getting it out. This happens smoothly and baby is fine – and will continue to be until it gets home schooled and taken on all-naked, yurt-based family holidays. A

---

* 'Cholelithoproctophilia' would be shoving gallstones up your arse, but I've just made it up. 'Orbitobelonephilia' – sticking needles in your eyes. 'Craniophallic anastamosis' – dickhead.

couple of minutes later, I'm delivering the placenta and look up to have the awkward discussion about what GL would like me to do with it. She has a kidney dish in her hands and is shovelling handfuls of blood clots into her mouth.

'Isn't *this* the placenta?' she asks, blood dribbling out of the corner of her mouth like the disgusting progeny of Dracula and the Cookie Monster. I explain that it's just some clots I left in a bowl after delivering baby. She turns ashen, then green. Clearly blood isn't the delicious post-delivery snack she imagines placenta might be. She holds up the kidney dish and vomits into, onto and around it. Sorry, I mean experiences haematemesis.

Wednesday, 19 September 2007

Email from Head of Administration, Undergraduate Learning Centre:

> *Dear Adam,*
>
> *As you know, we are grateful for your commitment to undergraduate teaching. In future when emailing the fourth-year students about teaching sessions, kindly refer to the Undergraduate Learning Centre as the Undergraduate Learning Centre, not the Early Learning Centre.*

Tuesday, 2 October 2007

Retrieve my phone from the locker after an unremitting day on labour ward. Seven missed calls from Simon and a bunch of voicemails, all from this morning. I hesitate before pressing play – I know in my heart it'll be too late already; I'm already half preparing what to say to the coroner. Turns out Simon's pocket-dialled me, the little bastard.

Wednesday, 24 October 2007

It's a quiet night on labour ward so I go to my on-call room, lie in bed and piss around on Facebook for a bit. Someone has linked to a bucket list quiz, where you tick off, from a checklist of 100, various things you've achieved in your life. Have you visited the Great Wall of China? Ridden an ostrich? Been eaten out by one of Barry Manilow's security team in a Las Vegas infinity pool? It turns out I've done very few things at all. I check my emails, then have a wank.*

Mid-wank, the crash bleep† goes off. Scrub trousers back on, I rush into a delivery room – the mother is

---

* I don't know what the GMC position is regarding wanking in on-call rooms. An email to them asking for clarification sat unsent in my drafts folder for over a month when I was putting this book together, before I chickened out and deleted it. But we've all done it. Basically, make sure your doctor uses the hand gel when he rushes into your room at night.

† For life or death emergencies, you can be summoned by a 'crash

pushing and there's an extremely worrying CTG. Within a minute of walking into the room I have delivered the baby by forceps extraction. Mother and baby both fine, good old me. I can now write my own bucket list and tick off 'Delivered a baby while still erect'.

Thursday, 1 November 2007

I've barely started an emergency caesarean when my SHO bursts into theatre to tell me that a patient in another room has a non-reassuring trace and might need an instrumental delivery. My senior registrar is performing some complicated and repulsive emergency gynae op in main theatre and this SHO is a GP trainee on a six-month placement, so it's my show entirely. I get her to take a photo of the CTG on her phone so I can see how bad it is and attempt to construct some sort of a plan.

By the time she pops back to theatre, I've delivered the baby and am starting to sew up the uterus. The trace is much worse than the SHO described, and I have another fifteen minutes of needlework still to go. I put in another stitch to stop the uterus bleeding and ask the scrub nurse to rest a large wet swab over the patient's open abdomen (leaving her looking like a horrendous Tellytubby) then make my apologies and run off to perform a quick forceps delivery on the other baby. I've

---

bleep' – your bleep is granted the power of speech and tells you exactly where to run to, saving valuable seconds.

barely got the tongs off its head when the emergency buzzer blares from the room next door. Another grotty trace, this time needing a ventouse extraction, then management of a post-partum haemorrhage afterwards for good measure.

By the time I get back to theatre to polish off my original caesarean it's nearly ninety minutes later, and when *that* one's done, it's time to hand over to the morning registrar. I tell him my tale of super-heroism, expecting him to suggest they rename the hospital after me. All I get in reply is a 'yeah, that happens', like I've mentioned the coffee shop has run out of pains aux raisins.

Monday, 5 November 2007

Patient in antenatal clinic told me she was taking Dorothy every morning because she was feeling stressed. Who's Dorothy? Some great aunt she was escorting down to the shops as a strange kind of chill-out exercise, like a mental health assistance dog? She informed me Dorothy was the street name for ketamine.[*]

'Does it help with the stress?' I asked – and was genuinely interested in the answer.

---

[*] Other terms for ketamine include K, Kit Kat and Special K. Although if she'd told me she was having Special K every morning I may well have missed the reference.

Monday, 12 November 2007

All surgical staff have been summoned to the Early Learning Centre for a lecture on patient safety. Last week a patient had their completely healthy left kidney removed, leaving them only with a completely useless right kidney.

We're reminded that in the last three years, neurosurgeons in this country have drilled holes in the wrong side of patients' skulls fifteen times. Fifteen times they couldn't tell left from right with a Black and Decker at your bonce. Feels like grounds for retiring the 'it's hardly brain surgery' maxim.

The hospital is very keen mistakes like the great kidney snafu aren't repeated – although it's slightly too late for this poor guy, whose ashes have presumably just been scattered on the wrong beach.

The upshot is that new hospital protocol states any patient going to theatre must have a large arrow drawn in Sharpie pen on their left or right leg as appropriate. I put my hand up and ask what happens if the patient already has a tattoo of an arrow on the wrong leg. Decent laugh from the lecture theatre and my consultant calls me a fucking clown.

Tuesday, 13 November 2007

I receive an email from Dr Vane, Director of Clinical Governance, advising that if a patient has a tattoo of an arrow on either leg, then it should be covered up with Micropore tape and a new arrow drawn in Sharpie on the correct leg. This will now be included in the policy document, and he thanks me for my valuable contribution.

Tuesday, 8 January 2008

The population is getting fatter faster than a mobility scooter hurtling towards Greggs at closing time. Today our labour ward operating table is being replaced for the second time in as many years, because last month a woman exceeded the weight capacity for the recently acquired 'obese table'.

I realize it's a complicated issue, but surely being so big that special equipment has to be ordered in for you would be the first clue that now would be a good time to offload some timber.

The even newer table has enormous wings that flap up from the sides to prevent 'overspill', like an industrial version of the dinner table that grandma can extend at Christmas to fit on all the extra vol-au-vents. I reckon you could comfortably rest the *Cutty Sark* on it – it took ten men, some hydraulic equipment and the best part of two hours to get it into theatre. I presume the next issue will be the table crashing through the floor one day mid-caesarean, killing the entire dermatology department beneath us.

Saturday, 19 January 2008

Today I tipped into full-blown Stockholm Syndrome and decided to go into work on a Saturday off. 'If you're having an affair you can just tell me, you know,' H said.

I performed my first TAH BSO* yesterday and wanted to check the patient was doing OK. Every time my phone buzzed this morning I assumed it was a message from the weekend team to tell me her wound had exploded or I'd punctured her bowel, severed a ureter or let her quietly bleed to death internally. I basically just needed a bit of reassurance to stop myself going insane.

Obviously, she was absolutely fine, and had already been reviewed by my colleague Fred. I immediately felt bad – I'd hate him to think I didn't trust him to do his job properly (which I don't), so I nimbly hurried off the ward in order to escape unnoticed. Or not so nimbly – I bumped into him on my way out and had to pretend I was 'just passing by', so thought I'd check she was OK.

'Don't blame you,' Fred said, shrugging, and told me his first major op died in hospital. He'd reviewed her obsessively and planned her post-op care meticulously. Then, on the day she was meant to go home, she choked to death on an egg and cress sandwich.

---

* Total abdominal hysterectomy and bilateral salpingo-oophorectomy is the removal of the uterus, cervix, tubes and ovaries. Salpingo-oopherectomy has three 'o's in a row, which has to be some kind of record?

I'm now half considering making my patient nil-by-mouth until discharge, just to be on the safe side. Having 'just passed by', I begin the hour-long drive back home and think about what H said earlier. Even if I wanted to have an affair, I honestly think I'd be too tired to unzip my trousers.

Tuesday, 26 February 2008

About to perform a hysteroscopy* on patient FR and as I'm talking through the procedure, she asks, 'What's the worst that could happen?' Patients ask this all the time, and I wish they wouldn't because obviously the truthful answer is they could die. In her case, as with almost everyone who asks this, the chances of death are infinitesimal, but the question forces my hand into name-checking the Reaper immediately before their operation.

For the past few months, whenever someone has asked, 'What's the worst that could happen?' I've replied, 'The world could explode.' This generally has the effect of making the patient realize they're catastrophizing, and breaks the ice a little. Plus, it's not a lie – one day it will, and doubtless I'll be working on labour ward when it does.

---

* Putting a camera inside the uterus. One of the mainstays of gynaecology investigations – principally for abnormal bleeding, but also a traditional procedure if you don't really know what else to do. The procedure was first performed in 1869, and most units haven't bought new equipment since.

On this occasion, FR is a fervent believer that the world *is* going to end in the next five years and invites me to a David Icke[*] lecture at Brixton Academy next week. I might even go. What's the worst that could happen?

Friday, 29 February 2008

Special occasions tend to call for patients to insert special types of object into their vaginas and recta. Christmas in particular has rewarded me well, with a stuck fairy ('Do you want it back?' 'Yeah, bit of a rinse and she'll be grand'), a grossly swollen vulva from a mistletoe contact allergy and mild vaginal burns from a patient stuffing a string of lights inside and turning them on (bringing new meaning to the phrase 'I put the Christmas lights up myself'). This is my first leap year working as a doctor and the Great British public have pulled it out of the bag for me with a very, very specific injury.

Patient JB decided to take advantage of tradition and propose to her boyfriend – going to the expense of buying an engagement ring, the trouble of putting it inside a Kinder Surprise egg and the imagination of inserting it vaginally. She would suggest some finger-work to her partner, he would discover it, retrieve it and

---

[*] Icke is a professional conspiracy theorist and Holocaust denier, who puts on inexorably long, mad speeches. By the time this book is published he'll no doubt be foreign secretary.

then she would go down on one knee (and, presumably, him). Equal parts unexpected, disgusting and, I suppose, romantic. Unfortunately, he was unable to retrieve it as planned – it had rotated itself lengthwise – and no amount of shoogling from either of them would get this particular goose to lay her golden egg. Remarkably, she was so keen to maintain the surprise she wouldn't tell him what she'd done or why, but eventually decided this was a hospital matter, so we met in cubicle three. It was a very easy delivery with a pair of sponge-holding forceps.

She hadn't told me about the contents of the egg either at this point, so there was a moment of confusion for both me and the boyfriend when she asked him to open it. I gave him a pair of latex gloves, sandblasting the very last pico-trace of romance from the scenario. She popped the question and he said yes; presumably out of shock, or fear of what a woman who does that with a Kinder Surprise would do to him if spurned. I wonder where the best man will keep the wedding bands during the ceremony?

Monday, 17 March 2008

I'm unsure who decided that junior doctors have so much spare time on our hands that we should conduct annual audits, but the audit meeting is this week, so I'm sitting reviewing patient notes after my night shift, going through the motions like Lady Chatterley in her marriage to the cockless Sir Clifford. As well as collecting my official audit data on APGAR scores* I have spotted an interesting incidental finding, and have put together some data on that too.

Introduction
2,500 babies are delivered annually on our unit, of which roughly 750 are caesarean sections. The surgeon records hand-written operation notes for every patient, representing the permanent legal record of the procedure.

Methods
I personally reviewed the operative notes of 382 caesarean sections, representing all such procedures performed between January and June 2007.

Results
In 109 cases (28.5 per cent) the surgeon performing the procedure has misspelled 'caesarean' as 'caesarian'.

Conclusion
In almost a third of cases, my colleagues are idiots and can't spell the name of the only fucking operation they have to remember the name of.

---

* APGAR scores are the standard measure of how well a newborn baby is doing – they get marks for Appearance, Pulse, Grimace, Activity and Respiration. It was devised by a doctor called Virginia Apgar, which makes me think she chose arbitrary measures just because they fitted with her surname. Like if I decided that the best measures of a baby's health were Kicking, Applauding and Yawning.

Thursday, 17 April 2008

Sometimes it's the little things that make a difference on labour ward. The touch on your arm and a muttered thank you from the mum too exhausted by her labour to speak. The Diet Coke an SHO buys you because you look so knackered. The reassuring nod from your consultant that says 'you've got this'. And sometimes it's the really massive things that make a difference – like a patient's husband taking me to one side after an emergency caesarean to thank me, mentioning that he's head of marketing for the UK operations of a large champagne house and taking my name so he can send me 'a little something'. I spend a week dreaming of splashing about in a gigantic champagne coupe filled to the brim with prohibitively expensive fizz, like an ostentatious burlesque act.

Today a package arrived for me at work – and I don't mean to be ungrateful, but seriously? A branded baseball cap and key ring?

Monday, 21 April 2008

Performing an elective caesarean section, assisted by a hungover medical student. With the possible exception of diathermy,* which smells deliciously like frying bacon,

---

* Diathermy is essentially a soldering iron – it heats up the area you touch it on and stops small blood vessels from bleeding by sealing them off. It is important not to clean the skin with alcohol-based

the sights and smells of labour ward theatres aren't great for the morning after. Take a look at the ingredients: there's over half a litre of blood spilled, plus a tidal wave of amniotic fluid when you cut through the uterus, the baby's covered in more gunk than you'd find in the plughole of a cattery and the placenta always smells like stale semen – none of which you really want to be faced with when your burps still taste of Jägerbomb and you're sweating rogan josh through your eyeballs. Baby delivered, and just as I was sewing up the uterus, the student fainted, face-planting right into the open abdomen. 'We should probably give the patient some antibiotics,' the anaesthetist suggested.

Tuesday, 13 May 2008

At a pub quiz with Ron and a few others and one of the questions is 'How many bones are there in the human body?' I'm out by about sixty, to the general outrage of my teammates. I try to explain myself: it's not something you'd ever be taught; there's no clinical situation where you'd actually need to know this; it's an irrelevance; I wouldn't expect Ron to be able to say how many types of tax there are . . . But it's too late. I can see from the look on everyone's horrified faces that they're trying to think back to all the times they've asked for medical

---

antiseptic before the operation, otherwise diathermy sparks can set the patient on fire.

advice from a doctor who doesn't even know how many bones there are. Three other teams got the correct answer.*

Monday, 2 June 2008

Antenatal clinic. Called in by a midwife to review her patient – a low-risk primip† at thirty-two weeks, here for a routine check-up. The midwife was unable to pick up baby's heart with the Sonicaid‡ so wants me to pop in. This happens fairly often, and 99 per cent of the time all is well. I tend to grab a portable ultrasound machine, wheel it in like a hostess trolley, quickly show the parents their baby's heart on a monitor and then wheel it all back out again, grinning like a gameshow compère. When they've had the agony of listening in vain for baby's heart swoosh-swooshing, all they want is some unequivocal evidence on a screen.

This is clearly the 1 per cent though, and I can tell as soon as I enter the room. This midwife really knows what she's doing, and she looks ashen. The patient is a GP, married to an ophthalmology registrar, so we're in the rare situation where everyone in the room already

---

* It's 206.

† Primip (short for primiparous), meaning first pregnancy. Multip (multiparous) for subsequent pregnancies.

‡ Sonicaid is the handheld device that you listen for babies' hearts with.

knows there's something seriously wrong. I can't even manage my 'I'm sure everything's fine' speech before I put the ultrasound probe on.

To make matters worse, I have to call a consultant in to confirm fetal death for the notes, even though both parents know I've been looking at the four unmoving chambers of their baby's heart on the screen. She's being rational, practical, collected – suddenly in work mode, her emotional shields up as high as mine. He's in bits. 'You shouldn't have to bury your child.'

Thursday, 5 June 2008

The rota has been flinging me around the hospital seemingly at random – from antenatal clinic to gynae theatre to infertility clinic to labour ward to colposcopy to scanning – so everyone feels like a stranger at the moment. I've all but given up hope of seeing someone I recognize, unless they're handing me a latte in Costa.

It's especially rare to see the same patient more than once, but on my afternoon round of labour ward I see the GP I'd diagnosed with an intra-uterine death in clinic earlier this week. She's now in labour, having been induced.* She and her husband seem oddly pleased to see me – a familiar face, someone who doesn't need an

---

* It's a terrible cruelty that if a baby dies in utero, the safest place to deliver is on labour ward, surrounded by dozens of mothers and babies.

explanation and is already tuned in to what's happening, can be of some comfort on such an awful, scary day.

What the hell can you say? It feels like a woeful gap in our training that no one's ever told us about talking to grieving couples. Will I make it better or worse if I talk positively about 'next time'? I want to give them hope, but feel like I shouldn't say it. It's an extreme version of 'there are plenty more fish in the sea' after a break-up, as if babies are totally interchangeable, just so long as you have one. Do I say how sad I feel for them? Is that making it all about me, giving them yet another person's feelings to consider? They'll have plenty of their own family members throwing themselves at their feet in misery; they certainly don't need this from me. How about a hug? Too much? Not enough?

Stick to what you know. I just talk practically about what will happen over the next few hours. They have a thousand questions, which I answer as best I can. This is clearly their way of coping for now, medicalizing it.

I pop back every hour or so to see how they're doing. It goes past 8 p.m., and I decide to stay on labour ward until they've delivered. H is expecting me back home any minute but I lie in a text that there's been an emergency and I need to stay. I don't know why I can't just tell the truth. I lie to the patient too when she asks why I'm still here gone 11 p.m. 'I'm covering for someone,' I say. It does feel like my presence, if not my conversational skills, are helping them a bit.

Delivery happens shortly after midnight, and I take

blood samples from mum and talk through all the possible tests we can do to find a cause for the stillbirth. They opt for everything, which is understandable, but this means I have to take skin and muscle samples from baby, the worst thing for me in this whole job. It used to upset me so much when I first started that I'd practically have to look away while I did the necessary. Now, slightly more desensitized to a thing you can never quite believe you'll ever become desensitized to, I can look. I just find it heartbreakingly sad cutting into a dead baby. We expect them to look beautiful, perfect, unspoiled; often they don't. He's been dead a couple of weeks, looking at him – he's macerated, skin peeling, head softened, almost burnt-looking. 'I'm sorry,' I say to him as I take the samples I need. 'There we go, all done now.'

I dress him again, look up to a God I don't believe in and say, 'Look after him.'

Tuesday, 10 June 2008

Stopped by the police in Holland Park. 'Did you know you just ran a red light there, sir?' I honestly didn't. I'd been driving home on autopilot, utterly exhausted after a relentless night shift that included five caesarean sections. Hopefully I was paying more attention in theatre than on the road.

I explain to my frontline brothers that I've just come off labour ward after thirteen hours. They give not a single shit, a £60 fine and three penalty points.

Wednesday, 18 June 2008

I'm no stranger to speaking in code in front of patients. Just a stray word here or there can be the difference between a patient drawing up ambitious plans to build a shrine in your honour and hysterically accusing you of plotting their demise. So we've got our equivalent of spelling out W-A-L-K-I-E-S in front of the dog or T-R-I-A-L S-E-P-A-R-A-T-I-O-N to fox an eavesdropping five-year-old.* But it's not just patients who need to be kept in the dark from time to time. On this job I've also had to develop a code so Miss Bagshot can't understand me,

---

* There are three grades of code. Firstly, there's the formal Latin and Greek terms for conditions. So, we say 'dyspnoea' rather than 'shortness of breath' and 'epididymo-orchitis' rather than 'gammy cock and balls'. Secondly, there's using a layer of euphemism. Instead of suggesting syphilis, we ask to 'check the VDRL', which is the lab test involved; rather than saying HIV, we can talk about 'CD4 deficiency', referring to the underlying immune problem. Thirdly, and much more fun, are the completely made-up ones that have entered medical vocab in the last couple of decades. They generally sound credible and scientific, and allow you to be frank in front of the patient without them realizing.

A few of my favourites are:

Chronic glucose poisoning – Obesity.

Incarceritis – Onset of symptoms immediately following arrest.

Q sign – Tongue hanging out of side of mouth, in the shape of a Q. Prognostically-speaking, a very bad sign, though not as bad as the Dotted Q sign, where there's a fly on the tongue.

Status dramaticus – Medically well but over-emotional.

Therapeutic phlebotomy – Gets better after a blood test.

Transferred to the fifteenth floor – Dead. (NB The number should be one higher than number of floors in the hospital.)

just to survive her interminable consultant ward rounds. When I need a caffeine hit I tell the house officer to 'review Mrs Buckstar', and he pops down to Starbucks for me. Three months in and she hasn't broken this seemingly uncrackable cipher. Either that or she's turned on by my coffee breath.

Friday, 20 June 2008

I'm teaching the SHO a method of skin closure using staples that I think gives as good a cosmetic result as sutures in a quarter of the time.* He does an excellent job using this technique, but I count at the end that he has used ten staples. I explain it's bad luck to close with an even number of staples and ask him to put in an extra one in the middle of the incision. I'm not superstitious – I'll happily limbo under ladders or live in a flat full of open umbrellas – but it's something I was taught years ago and have passed on to juniors ever since. Science may trump the supernatural, but once someone tells you an operative technique is bad luck, it's probably better to be safe than sorry. No one wants to be bleeped in the middle of the night because a plateful of intestines have made a surprise appearance out the front of a patient's abdomen.

---

* Materials and technique in skin closure vary surgeon by surgeon. The staplers, and indeed staples, used are a barely modified version of the kind you'd buy at Rymans.

Fully briefed on how to fend off this imminent crisis from the spirit world, my SHO takes the staple gun to insert the final talisman – and accidentally drives a staple deep into the pulp of my finger.

Thursday, 3 July 2008

Patient TH has been telling me for two days now that her breast pump is bugged. I've had to promise her that we'll have it investigated because when I tried to reassure her initially, she started screaming that I was in with the Russians as well. I made my fairly uncontroversial diagnosis of puerperal psychosis,* but failed to persuade the psychiatrists that she was sufficiently unhinged to justify a review. They weren't convinced she was at risk of endangering herself or her baby. It felt rather like an orthopaedic team refusing to see a patient who had a broken leg on the basis they weren't due to participate in the New York Marathon.

Phone call from A&E today – patient TH is currently being reviewed by psychiatry having been brought in by the police. The Starbucks downstairs had phoned 999 after she rocked up, stripped off all her clothes, stood on a table and started singing 'Holding out for a Hero'. Useful to know where the psychiatrists set the bar.

---

* Puerperal psychosis is the nuclear version of postnatal depression – severe psychiatric symptoms in the days after giving birth, occurring in roughly 1 in 1,000 women.

Friday, 4 July 2008

Patient NS presents to urogynae clinic for replacement of a lost ring pessary.* She asks if there are options other than the ring type, because they have a bit of 'baggage' for her now. She's fifty-eight years old, and a few weeks ago was dancing at her niece's wedding, wearing 'less than substantial' underwear beneath her dress. Her vigorous Macarena-ing caused the pessary to dislodge and plunge straight down onto the dance floor then happily roll across it, eventually coming to a halt at the feet of the best man.

'What's this?' he bellowed, holding it aloft. 'Has someone's pram lost a wheel? Oh! Is it some kid's teething ring?' The patient departed the dance floor and the wedding before she found out whether or not it got thrust into some poor toddler's mouth. I offer her a shelf pessary† and a sympathetic smile.

---

* A ring pessary is a doughnut of stiff plastic that goes up your vagina and keeps your internal organs, well, internal. Pessaries have existed as long as pelvic organ prolapse, which is to say a couple of years after the first woman gave birth. Historically, a popular type of pessary was the potato – shove it up there and everything stays put nicely. Horrifyingly, the warm and moist environment is an ideal sprouting environment for root vegetables, so they would have to trim the green shoots as soon as they started bristling against their underwear.

† A shelf pessary looks like one of those hooks you put on the back of your bedroom door to hang your dressing gown on. You get it in or out by holding the hook bit, and the plate section keeps your uterus out of the public eye.

Monday, 7 July 2008

Crash call to a labour ward room. The husband was dicking around on a birthing ball and fell off, cracking his skull on the ground.

Tuesday, 8 July 2008

The phrase 'rollercoaster of emotions' gets a lot of air-time in obs and gynae but I've never seen the big dipper hurtle round its loop quite as fast as today. Called to the Early Pregnancy Unit by one of the SHOs to confirm a miscarriage at eight weeks – he's new to scanning and wants a second pair of eyes. I remember that feeling only too well and scamper over. He's managed the couple's expectations very well, and clearly made them aware it doesn't look good – they're sad and silent as I walk in.

What he hasn't done very well is the ultrasound. He may as well have been scanning the back of his hand or a packet of Quavers. Not only is the baby fine, but so is the other baby that he hadn't spotted. Not sure I've ever had to break *good* news before.[*]

---

[*] Twins occur in 1 in 80 spontaneous pregnancies – they're more common in IVF because you generally implant a couple of embryos a pop. Chances of triplets are 1 in 80 squared (1:6,400), quads are 1 in 80 cubed (1:512,000) and so on. Almost every complication of pregnancy is more likely the more babies you're carrying – anything higher-order than twins is generally a bit of an obstetric catastrophe.

Thursday, 10 July 2008

Next week me and H head off for a fortnight in Mauritius, to celebrate five years together. I'm excited about a bleep-free existence and hopeful I haven't forgotten how to have a relationship that isn't conducted over hurried breakfasts and apologetic texts.

The problem with being in a bubble is that it only takes one prick to burst it. It comes in the form of an email from medical staffing, letting me know I now need to work the middle weekend. None of my colleagues can swap with me and I don't know how to deliver babies over Skype, so I go back to medical staffing to explain my predicament. I have the kind of sinking feeling you'd have going to the headmaster's office to deny you stole liquorice from the tuck shop, with teeth stained carbon-black.

I know colleagues who've had to cut honeymoons short and miss family funerals, so the odds were never great for them bending the rota for a holiday. They refuse to organize a locum – their best suggestion is that I pop back to England for a bit. I don't think I'll get away with breaking this one to H by text message.

Although I once had a patient with quads, and I seem to remember she ended up getting free nappies, clothes, baby food and a people carrier by way of sponsorship.

6

Registrar – Post Two

I would always feel tremendously proud to say that I worked for the NHS – who doesn't love the NHS? (Well, apart from the Secretary of State for Health.) It's unlike any other national asset; no one talks in fond tones about the Bank of England or would think any less of you if you suggested suing Cardiff Airport. It's easy to work out why: the NHS does the most amazing job and we've all benefitted from it. They delivered you when you were born and one day they'll zip you up in a bag, but not until they've done everything that medical science will allow to keep you on the road. From cradle to grave, just like your man Bevan promised back in 1948.

They fixed your broken arm on sports day, they gave your nan chemo, they treated the chlamydia you brought back from Kavos, they started you on that inhaler, and all this wizardry was free at the point of service. You don't have to check your bank balance after booking an appointment: the NHS is always there for you.[*]

---

[*] For now, at least.

On the other side of the fence, knowing you were working for the NHS took the sting out of so many things about the job: the vicious hours, the bureaucracy, the understaffing, the way they inexplicably blocked Gmail on all the computers in one hospital I worked at (thanks, guys!). I knew I was part of something good, important, irreplaceable, and so I did my bit. I don't have an amazing inbuilt work ethic, it's not applied to anything I've ever done since (as my publisher will attest), but the NHS is something special, and the alternative is horrifying.

We should see the skyscraper-high bills of America as the ghost of Christmas future when it comes to NHS privatization. Politicians may act dumb, but they're not, and we'll be lured very stealthily into this particular gingerbread house. We'll be promised it's only little corners of the NHS that are changing, but there'll be no trail of breadcrumbs to help us find our way back through the forest. One day you'll blink and the NHS will have completely evaporated – and if that blink turns out to be a stroke then you're totally screwed.

My opinion of private healthcare in the UK changed a bit during my time as a registrar. I used to be on board with it, seeing it as much like private schooling: a bunch of rich people who save the taxpayer a few quid by going off and doing their own thing, no harm done. I could always see myself doing the odd bit of private work as a consultant – one evening a week in clinic maybe, the occasional hysteroscopy list if I thought I deserved a Mercedes, perhaps a caesarean a month if I thought my Mercedes deserved a chauffeur. I knew consultants who had this life, and it didn't hurt my motivation to imagine it for myself.

And then in my second year as a registrar I started doing regular locum work. I'd rather overstretched myself on the mortgage and it felt like a sensible way of making my income do at least a reasonable impression of my outgoings. As free time was in short supply (and what I had of it didn't just feel like *mine* to give away), I generally took night shifts sandwiched between normal days at work and, in order to guarantee an hour or two of sleep, I would do them in private hospitals or private wings of NHS hospitals, where the workload is a lot lighter.

These days I get asked fairly often by friends who've made much better life choices than me about whether they should have their baby privately. These are people who order from the bottom of the wine list to get a better wine, or order from the bottom of the holiday home in the Chilterns list to get a better holiday home in the Chilterns. People who know that while money might not buy you happiness, it certainly buys you nicer stuff.

This theory, it turns out, doesn't really work with childbirth. It's a shame, because if you choose to go private you'll be spunking around fifteen grand on it, and it won't be covered by your health insurance. You'll definitely get a nicer hospital room and nicer food.

You'll certainly get an elective caesarean if you ask for one. In fact, your consultant might actively encourage you to have one. They can bill you extra for it on top of the fifteen grand – plus they know they won't get unexpectedly bleeped in the middle of a dinner party to pull a baby out of you. And if you start to bleed a few hours later, when your consultant is back home, the resident doctor will run along. When it was me, fine – I could deal with it, it was my day job. But I could see the rest of the rota; and a lot of my colleagues in private-locum-land normally worked as SHOs, some of them extremely junior ones, and would be woefully under-equipped to deal with a situation like that.

But what if there's a major emergency, beyond any single doctor's capabilities? One where you need a team of obstetricians, anaesthetists, paediatricians, maybe even medics and surgeons from other specialities? Then all you can do is call 999, have your patient taken to an NHS unit designed to cope with this scenario and hope they live long enough to get there.

You can google the names of private maternity units alongside the words 'out of court settlement' if you want case studies. As I say, the food's always excellent. Whether it's to die for is your decision.

Personally, I didn't ever want to risk being the doctor holding the ball when it all went wrong, so I bailed on private medicine after a few months of these shifts. Which was a bit of a shame as I'd already decided what colour uniform my chauffeur would wear.

Saturday, 9 August 2008

Non-medic friends are always impressed when I perform spot diagnoses on members of the public – like an advanced level of 'I Spy'. The lady on the bus with early Parkinson's, the man at the restaurant with lipodystrophy from HIV medication, the guy with the eye changes denoting high cholesterol, the characteristic flapping hand of liver disease, the fingernail changes of lung cancer.

But there's clearly a time and a place. 'Trichomonas Vaginalis,' I say proudly, pointing out the telltale green discharge residue on the stripper's vulva. And just like that, I'm ruining the stag do, apparently.

Monday, 11 August 2008

Moral maze. On a locum shift in a unit with some private labour ward rooms, and called in by the midwife to see a woman who is pushing and has a worrying trace. I let the patient know I need to give her baby a hand coming out because its heart rate has dropped quite a bit. I tell her there's no time to wait for her consultant to come in, but it's literally my bread and butter, and everything will be absolutely fine. She understands.

Out of the room I call her consultant, Mr Dolohov,

a traditional courtesy with a private patient. He isn't very courteous in response. He says he's only a minute away and coming straight over: under no circumstances am I to deliver 'his' patient. I go back into the room and prepare everything for his arrival – forceps, delivery pack, suture set. And then I decide this is ridiculous; the baby is clearly unwell and will deteriorate every moment I don't deliver it. What if he's only a minute away like every minicab is 'only a minute away'? If the baby comes out compromised because of my inaction, that's my GMC number up the fuck. And worse, it's a damaged baby. If this Mr Dolohov wants to complain about me, the worst that can happen is I never work again in a hospital I now have no desire to work in.

I deliver the baby – it takes a moment to breathe but soon perks up, and cord gases* confirm I was right not to wait. I deliver the placenta, stitch up a graze, clean up the patient and say, 'Adam's a good name.' She's calling it Barclay, naturally. Still no consultant. Moral maze correctly navigated.

I've already got changed into fresh scrubs by the time Mr Dolohov finally appears. To give him credit, he's heard the cord gases from a midwife and gives me a huge apology. I'd have preferred it if he'd given me a huge sum

---

* After the baby is born and handed over to the paediatricians, you take a sample of blood from the bit of umbilical cord attached to the placenta, known as 'cord gases'. They get tested on a machine on labour ward and definitively show how urgently the baby needed to have been delivered.

of money, especially as he'll be charging the patient thousands of pounds for the delivery that *I* did, but there you go.

Friday, 5 September 2008

'Do you have a place?' asked Mr Lockhart as I joined him in morning antenatal clinic. It took me a moment – we'd been talking about holidays, how I'd finally booked one and was off to France with H.

'Yes . . . I mean, we've booked our tickets . . .'

'No! A place! Do you have a little place there?'

How deliciously out of touch he was with the life of a registrar. I can barely afford the mortgage on a tiny flat despite our two incomes; a bolthole in France seems as likely a next move as buying a racehorse or a time-share on the Death Star. But on the other hand, this is clearly a normal thing for a consultant to have – an aspirational light at the end of the registrar tunnel.

He apologizes for the fact that he's going to have to leave clinic a little early today – in fact, he should prob-ably leave now. There are fifty-two patients in clinic and I'm now the only doctor here. There may well be a light at the end of the tunnel, but the tunnel is eighty-five miles long, crammed full of impacted faeces, and I have to eat my way out of it.

Thursday, 11 September 2008

I almost cry at the end of an unforgiving night shift when I see my pigeonhole has something other than a nit-picking memo about parking or hand gel; it's a lovely card from a patient. I remember her well. I repaired a tear she sustained a couple of weeks ago during a spontaneous vaginal delivery.

> *Dear Adam,*
>
> *Just wanted to say thank you. You did a fantastic job – my GP checked my stitches and said you could hardly tell I'd had a baby, let alone a third-degree tear! I'm extremely grateful to you. Thank you again.*

Everything about it is so thoughtful, the kind of thing that makes the whole job totally worthwhile. She'd even made it herself – beautiful textured white card adorned with her baby's footprint in gold paint on the front. Then again, I guess she didn't have much choice – there can't be much call in Paperchase for 'Thanks for mending my anus!' cards.

Tuesday, 16 September 2008

In labour ward triage a woman is furious that three or four people who arrived after her have been seen *before* her. 'If I ever have to go to hospital, madam,' one of the midwives calmly tells her, 'I want to be seen last. Because that means everyone else there is sicker than me.'

Thursday, 18 September 2008

My phone rings at 8 p.m. I try to guess whether it's because I've forgotten to turn up for a night shift or someone else has failed to turn up for one and I'm about to get pulled back to the ward on my invisible bungee rope. Happily, it's just my friend Lee, although he sounds rather worried. Lee is reliably my calmest, least flappable friend, so it's alarming to say the least. He works as a criminal defence lawyer, and I regularly hear him talking on the phone with policemen, judges and the like, cheerily asking, 'And was the whole body destroyed by the acid or just the skull?' or 'Roughly what size of genocide are we talking?' He asks if I'm free to come over; his flatmate Terry has injured himself and Lee suspects he may benefit from going to hospital, but would value my advice. It's not far away and I'm not doing anything that can't wait, so I pop over.

Terry has indeed injured himself. From the most insignificant of actions can come the most serious of consequences – and we've gone full 'butterfly effect' here. He cut his thumb opening a humble can of beans, has severed a little artery that's currently irrigating the floor and the top of his thumb is flapping open like a Muppet's mouth. There's even bone visible. I'm happy to provide my professional assessment that a visit to hospital is not just advised, but is both crucial and urgent. I suspect very few people in the world would disagree with me on this point. Unfortunately, Terry is one of them.

Lee takes me into the kitchen for a moment. Terry will take quite some persuading to go to hospital – he drinks rather heavily and worries that any blood tests will show liver damage and lead to a cascade of investigations and misery he has no interest in. It would also explain why he was bleeding so heavily and why the expression 'blood is thicker than water' didn't seem to apply to him.[*]

I spend a short while trying to negotiate with Terry. I suggest the doctors will be too concerned with the fact half his thumb is hanging off to bother delving too far into anything else, but it's clearly not a fight I'm going to win. He won't even let me call an ambulance so they can come and assess him. I go back through to Lee to formulate a Plan B, while Terry ruins a couple more tea towels. Plan B comes quite easily. I'm a doctor, Lee's a lawyer; between us we can section Terry under the Mental Health Act on the basis that he's a risk to himself. Lee, clearly knowing rather more about the Mental Health Act than I do, points out that not only can we definitely not section a patient between us, but he

---

[*] Among the liver's many and confusing functions, it produces a whole load of clotting factors, meaning that liver failure causes defective clotting.

wouldn't be a candidate for it anyway, as he's completely competent* to make the decision not to go to hospital.

Lee has a Plan C, which is presented to me in the form of a small crate of medical supplies. A year ago he took a holiday in Uganda (who actually does this?) and the advice given to plucky travellers is to buy one of these kits before you leave and keep it with you while you're away. If you get hospitalized during the trip, they can use your equipment rather than theirs, and you'll protect yourself from some hospitals' slightly laissez-faire attitude to infection control and a dose of HIV.

Lee unseals the case, opens it out in front of me like a dodgy market trader and asks me if I have what I need to sew Terry back up. He clearly splashed out on the de-luxe package – there's probably enough kit in there to take out a lung. After a short while cooing over it like an auntie trying to find the hazelnut swirl in a box of Milk Tray, I select suture material, scissors, needle-holders, swabs and cleaning solution – the only thing missing is some local anaesthetic. Lee jokes that Terry can just bite down on a wooden spoon.

And so, five minutes later, I find myself operating on a remarkably up-for-it Terry at the kitchen table. I clean the wound, place some big deep stitches to try and stop

___

* A patient is competent to make a decision if they can be demonstrated to understand the information they're being presented with, retain that information and weigh up the pros and cons. Even if their decision is absolutely bananas.

the arterial bleeder, then start closing the thumb up in layers as soon as everything's dry. The pain quickly gets a bit much for Terry to tolerate and – eager to keep his screams to a minimum (if the neighbours pop in to check everything's OK, this will all take some explaining) – Lee hands him the wooden spoon. And it works remarkably well.

I soon close up the skin and am rather pleased with the cosmetic result. I'm not sure how receptive Terry is to my advice on wound care and removal of stitches, but I give it anyway while he shivers his thanks and reaches for a drink, resolving never to eat beans again. I quietly ask Lee about the medico-legal implications of the evening's events. He laughs and swiftly changes the subject, packing me off in a cab with a nice bottle of rum. (Presumably Terry's.)

On the way home, I realize Terry should probably have a few days of antibiotics, given the slightly back-street nature of the procedure. I call Lee to make sure he sends Terry to the GP in the morning. I apologize for not writing a private prescription, but it's against GMC guidance to prescribe for friends and family. I can hear Lee's eyes rolling over the phone line. 'I think that's the least of your worries here.'

Thursday, 16 October 2008

Handing over an extremely busy labour ward to a locum. We've been working flat-out all day, and it's not going to be a quiet night either. There are a couple of women likely to end up with sections, a couple more heading towards instrumental delivery, plus a busy triage and A&E referrals Jenga-ing up. I apologize profusely – busy shifts are twice as difficult when you're a locum and don't know the peculiarities of a hospital. I can sense there's all sorts of inner turmoil going on behind his eyes, but he says nothing.

I realize I may have made it sound a little too ghastly, so back-pedal slightly. 'Room five might deliver normally, actually, and I don't think there's anything too urgent in A&E just now, so . . .' This doesn't seem to have done the trick – he still looks terrified. He asks me in broken English if he's expected to do caesareans. I suspect he's asking whether the SHO he's on with can operate, and I explain that she's very junior. But, no, he's asking if he might have to do a caesarean tonight – he's never done one before.

I ready myself for the explanation of what is clearly a hilarious misunderstanding. Maybe he's meant to be working as a neurology registrar and has just turned up on the wrong ward, and our real locum – the one who can actually do what we need them to do – is just about to stroll in, blaming some confusing signage. Nope, this guy accepted a shift from the locum agency as an obstetric registrar and no one there or at the hospital bothered to ask whether he'd ever worked on a labour ward before.

I send him home and call the consultant to ask what

to do, knowing full well the answer involves me working another twelve hours for free.

Monday, 20 October 2008

Patient HT has absolutely nothing wrong with her, physically at least. She's had normal blood tests, normal swabs, a normal hysteroscopy and a normal laparoscopy. There's no gynaecological (or any other kind of logical) cause for the pelvic pain she describes, and she's had no benefit whatsoever from the myriad treatments we've tried.

She still insists it's gynae. 'I know my own body!' She even knows the exact treatment she would like – for us to remove all of her pelvic organs. I and various colleagues and bosses have explained at length that we don't think it will help her symptoms in the slightest – plus it would be a big operation that carries non-trivial risks, including the chance it would cause adhesions* and result in worsened pelvic pain. She's adamant it's the only answer 'as I've been saying all along', and won't contemplate any options other than ripping out all of her plumbing. Maybe she's run out of storage at home and just wants to clear some extra space?

---

* Adhesions are bands of internal scar tissue, caused by previous operations or sometimes infections. They can cause pain for the patient, and also make subsequent operations much harder by gunking together all the organs. It's not always perfectly laid out in there like steaks and sausages on an OCD barbecue, you know.

It falls to me to finally discharge her from clinic and refer her to the pain management service, who will eventually get her on anti-depressants. This doesn't go down well, and I get everything from 'I've paid taxes all my life!' to 'Call yourself a doctor?' plus a list of all the people she's going to complain to, from the chief executive of the hospital to her MP. I tell her I appreciate her frustrations, but I really think we've done all we can for now. She asks me for a second opinion and I tell her she's already seen a large number of our doctors, all of whom were of the same opinion.

'I'm not leaving here until I'm booked in for this operation,' she announces, hands folded in her lap, and she clearly means it. I don't have time to wait for Satan to put on gloves and a North Face jacket, so I decide to book her in for another appointment in a few weeks' time – throwing a colleague under the same bus I've just dodged the fare on. I've got no doubt she can, and will, waste this clinic's resources for another year or more.

Before I offer her this appointment, she screams, 'Why does no one take me seriously?!' then picks up a sharps bin* and throws it at my head. I yelp, duck and constrict my anus to a one millimetre bore. The bin hits the wall above my desk and a shower of virulent needles

---

* Every office has separate bins for general rubbish, paper, plastics, etc., for everyone to ignore. In medical settings we also have the sharps bin – rigid plastic sweet tubs where you dispose of used needles, blades, lancets and the like.

rains down around me. Somehow, like Roadrunner escaping a Wile E. Coyote assassination attempt, they all miss me, and I avoid catching twelve strains of HIV. A nurse runs in to see what the kerfuffle is and then goes to phone security. And with that the patient is discharged from clinic. Next!

Thursday, 6 November 2008

I have lost a pen. Or more accurately, my pen has been stolen. Or even more accurately, it has been stolen by one of the three people in delivery room five: patient AG, her boyfriend or her mother. I wouldn't mind so much were it not a birthday present from H, were it not a Montblanc and had I not just delivered their baby.

The labour itself was without serious incident but they've been aggressive throughout my time with them and their feral snarling matched with the considerable tattoo count – baby excluded, for now – makes me slightly reluctant to accuse them of larceny.

I guess I'm lucky to have made it this many years without something getting pinched. Colleagues have had everything from scrub pockets picked, bags nicked from the nursing station and lockers broken into; not to mention tyres slashed in hospital car parks and even the odd physical assault.

I have a moan to Mr Lockhart, who I wouldn't trust to cut a patient's toenails, but is always good for a bit of advice and an anecdote. The advice was to forget it, don't get stabbed, and fair play to the patient for recognizing a decent pen. Then he got started on the anecdote.

Before his career in obs and gynae, Mr Lockhart worked as a GP in South London for a short chunk of the seventies. He celebrated getting a permanent job in general practice by buying himself a bright blue MGB convertible. The car was his pride and joy: he talked about it constantly to patients, friends and colleagues; waxed and polished it every weekend; only just stopped short of having a photo of it on his desk. And then one day it was over, as happens with all one-sided love affairs, when he finished surgery and clocked that the bright blue MGB convertible was missing from the surgery car park. He called the police, who did all they could, but ultimately failed to find the car. Lockhart's topic of conversation with patients, friends and colleagues now switched to the wretched state of the world – how could someone steal his beautiful car?

One day he was telling his tale of woe to a patient, who turned out to be a high-ranking member of what amounted to a local family of gangsters and, thanks to that bizarre moral code criminals seem to hold dear, was disgusted by this. What kind of lowlife would steal a doctor's car? Absolutely unacceptable. He said he was sure he'd be able to identify the felon and persuade them to return the car, though Mr L of course said there was absolutely no need – the same way you would claim there was 'absolutely no need' for someone to buy you an all-expenses-paid trip to the Seychelles. In other words, 'go on then'.

Later that week, Lockhart arrived at work to find a bright blue MGB convertible in the car park, its keys on the dashboard. His overwhelming relief turned to more mixed emotions at the realization that the car had a completely different number plate and interior.

Saturday, 15 November 2008

An email from Mme Mathieu telling me, with great regret, she's refunding the rest of the term's fee for my Conversational French class because I've now missed so many lessons it's pointless coming back. Email correspondence with Mme Mathieu is usually conducted entirely in French to fully immerse us in the language. This is the first email I've had from her in English; she's clearly not confident I'd understand otherwise, which really rubs *sel* into whatever the French for 'wound' is.

Monday, 17 November 2008

Superstition dictates you can't ever describe a shift as 'quiet'. Much like you don't say 'good luck' to an actor or 'go fuck yourself' to Mike Tyson. Say the Q word to a doctor and you're all but performing an incantation, summoning the sickest patients in the world to your hospital. I turn up for a locum night shift on a private obstetric unit and the registrar lets me know it should be 'very quiet tonight'. Before I have time to flick water at her and rattle off a few 'THE POWER OF CHRIST COMPELS YOU!'s she tells me a high-ranking royal from a Gulf state has just delivered a baby on labour ward, which goes some way to explaining the Oscars-level security everywhere and all the suede Ferraris outside.

As far as I'm concerned, roping off three tables in All Bar One for a twenty-first birthday is 'a bit swanky', but our esteemed guests have not only booked out the entire maternity unit so there's not a single other patient around, but their consultant will be staying overnight as well, just in case. It was fair to say the shift was quiet.

Tuesday, 18 November 2008

Ron phoned me for some medical advice this evening. His dad has been losing a lot of weight and having mid-chest discomfort and increasing difficulty in swallowing. When he went to his local surgery about it this morning, the GP thought he was looking a little yellow around the gills and referred him to be seen by gastro within the week. What did I think was going on?

If I was being asked on an exam paper, I'd have said it was metastatic oesophageal cancer with a survival rate of zero per cent. If I was being asked by a patient I'd have said it was very worrying and we'd want to investigate extremely urgently to rule out the possibility of cancer.

But if I'm asked by someone close to me? I said it sounded like his GP was doing everything right (true), and that it still could be nothing (definitely untrue – there was no plausible version of events where this was anything other than a very bad something). I desperately wanted it to be OK – for Ron and for his dad, who I've known since I was eleven – so I lied. You never lie to your patients to give them false hope, but there I was doing exactly that, reassuring my mate that everything would be fine.

We're constantly reminded by the GMC not to be doctor to friends or family, but I've always just ignored that and provided them an on-call private service. Because my job makes me such a useless friend in so many ways, I guess I feel like I have to offer *something* to justify my name on their Christmas card list. And this is basically why we're taught not to.

Thursday, 20 November 2008

In no other job would you be expected to wear shoes from a communal supply on a 'first come, first served' basis. It's like being at a Megabowl where people constantly get splashed with amniotic fluid, blood and placental tissue, and everyone's too lazy to clean them afterwards.

If you want your own personal white leather hospital clogs they cost around £80, so it's previously only consultants who've splurged on them, gliding around the hospital like they've got two giant paracetamols on their feet. But now there's a new breed of shoes called Crocs – they come in bright colours, do the same job and cost less than twenty quid. They have the added advantage of having holes in them, so you can padlock your pair together and no other bastard will get their hands or verrucas on them.

Today a notice has appeared in the changing rooms: 'Staff must under no circumstances wear Crocs footwear as the holes do not provide adequate protection from falling sharps.' A frustrated personal stylist has added underneath, 'And they make you look like a douche'.*

Saturday, 22 November 2008

Called to A&E to review a nineteen-year-old girl with heavy vaginal bleeding – same old, same old. What I'm in fact faced with is a nineteen-year-old girl who has taken kitchen scissors and performed her own labial reduction surgery. She valiantly managed to chop three-quarters of the way down her left labium minus before she called a) it a day, and b) an ambulance. It was an absolute mess down there, and bleeding heavily. I checked with my senior registrar that I wouldn't inadvertently be perform-ing female genital mutilation and go to prison if I cut off

---

* Presumably the same wag who changed the sign that says 'Warning! Thieves are operating in this department!' to 'Warning! Surgeons are operating in this department!'

the loose end and over-sewed the bleeding edge. All fine, and I tidied it up. In honesty, she didn't do much of a worse job than a lot of labiaplasties I've seen.

I booked her into gynae outpatients for a few weeks' time and we had a bit of a chat, emergency now out of the way. She told me she 'didn't think it would bleed', to which I didn't have anything to helpfully reply, and that she 'just wanted to look normal'. I reassured her there was absolutely nothing wrong with her labia; they really, honestly, did look normal. 'Not like in porn though,' she said.

There's been a lot of media noise about the damaging effects of porn and glossy magazines on body image, but this is the first time I've seen it first-hand – it's horrifying and depressing in equal parts. How long until we're seeing girls stapling their vaginas tighter?[*]

Wednesday, 10 December 2008

This week the hospital are running a diary card exercise.[†] I presume that in normal jobs they monitor employees

---

[*] The answer, as it turns out, was a year. A colleague saw a patient who'd superglued the introitus of her vagina because her boyfriend had been pressuring her to.

[†] During a diary card exercise, every doctor has to record their exact hours worked. But because the hospital can't (or don't want to) pay us for the time we actually work, they render the process completely meaningless. Either they lean on us to lie in the diary cards and just record our contracted hours or they throw dozens of consultants onto the wards to temporarily ease the burden on the juniors.

because staff are working *fewer* hours than they're paid for.

Consultants never previously spotted on a ward are seen writing discharge summaries for patients, working a few hours in labour ward triage, reviewing patients in A&E – to maximize the chance of the juniors leaving on time. This will continue until the nanosecond the diary card exercise ends, of course, but for now I'm enjoying the rewards. It's my third consecutive shift leaving on time, prompting H to sit me down and ask if I've been sacked.

To ensure the illusion of accuracy, clerical staff from hospital management shadow a few doctors at random during their shifts. I was joined by one on a night shift – or at least until 10.30 p.m. when she went home, unironically announcing she was exhausted.

Monday, 29 December 2008

Seeing a patient in gynae clinic whose GP recently started her on HRT patches and now has some PV bleeding. I ask her how long she's been on the HRT and she lifts up her blouse and counts the patches. 'Six . . . seven . . . eight weeks.' Her GP hadn't explained that she has to take the old ones off.

Saturday, 10 January 2009

Percy and Marietta's wedding today felt like a huge triumph against the odds. Not one, but two doctors able to get their big day off work. And the whole day too, not like my former colleague Amelia, who could only wangle the afternoon of her wedding day off, and ended up conducting her morning clinic in full hair and make-up to make the timings work.

The main miracle is they've managed to last this long together, despite a system seemingly designed to ruin their relationship. Percy and Marietta got their training posts in different deaneries, meaning the closest hospitals they could possibly work at over the course of five years were 120 miles apart. Rather than live together somewhere mutually inconvenient, Percy moved out to live in awful hospital accommodation and pop back home when the rota allowed, which it generally didn't.

In his speech, the best man, Rufus, a surgical trainee, compared their set-up to having a partner who works on the International Space Station. It was a brilliant speech, made all the more poignant because Rufus had to deliver it between the starter and main course. As soon as the pan-seared chicken livers were wolfed down, he had to dash off for a night shift.

Monday, 12 January 2009

Asked to review a patient in labour ward triage and repeat a PV as the midwife is uncertain of her findings. Her findings were of cephalic presentation with cervix 1 cm dilated. My findings are of breech presentation, cervix 6 cm dilated. I explain to mum that baby is bottom-down and the safest thing to do is to deliver by caesarean section. I don't explain to mum which part of the baby the midwife has just stuck her finger in to 1 cm dilatation.

Thursday, 22 January 2009

I accidentally dropped the on-call bleep into the labour ward macerator this evening, sending it off to a crunchy death. A feeling very similar to pissing your jeans – that wonderful warm sensation of enormous relief, followed almost immediately with, 'Fuck, what do I do now?!'

Thursday, 29 January 2009

Waited about a minute before making the uterine incision at caesarean until Heart FM had moved on to the next song. As appropriate as Cutting Crew may be for a surgeon, I refuse to deliver a baby to the refrain of 'I just died in your arms tonight'.

Friday, 30 January 2009

Patient DT is twenty-five years old and has attended colposcopy clinic* for her first smear test. And her second smear test: she has complete uterus didelphys –

---

* Colposcopy is a fancier way of doing smear tests – having a look at the neck of the womb for pre-cancer cells.

two vaginas, two cervices, two uteri. I've never seen this before. I perform both smears and spend a minute or two working out how the fuck to label the slides and forms, as the NHS cervical screening programme isn't really equipped for this admittedly rare scenario.

She's not seen a gynaecologist since she was a teenager so has a bunch of questions for me. I admit I've never come across a case like hers before, but answer the questions as best I can. She's mostly worried about future pregnancies.* I ask if she'd mind some questions in return. Potentially inappropriate, but we had a good rapport, and I'll probably never get the opportunity to chat to someone with the condition again.

Here's what I learned. She used to mention it to guys before they had sex, which tended to freak them out, so now she doesn't mention it at all. They apparently never notice in any case, which is hardly surprising – most guys' knowledge of female genital anatomy is sketchy at best. Aside from the old 'finding the clitoris' cliché, many don't seem to realize girls have a separate hole for peeing – they just think it's one great multi-functioning service tunnel. More than once I've catheterized a woman during labour only for her partner to ask if that isn't going to stop the baby from coming out.

---

* She's likely to be able to get pregnant, but there's increased chance of late miscarriage, premature birth, growth restriction and breech presentation, and she's much more likely to be delivered by caesarean.

The patient tells me she prefers having sex with her left vagina, as it's bigger (as I'd noted during examination – the right needed a smaller speculum), although she says it's nice to have an option for 'different sizes of guys'. I suggest that if she forgets which way round it is, the mnemonic 'righty tighty, lefty loosey' would apply – though in truth she's probably very unlikely to forget which way round her vaginas are.

I recount my tale to H after work. 'So it's like one of those metal pencil sharpeners at school with two sizes of hole?'

Tuesday, 3 February 2009

Last day at work before moving on to our next postings. It always feels odd to leave a job where you've watched lives begin and end, spent more hours than at your own house, seen the ward clerk more than your partner and have your departure go all but unacknowledged – but I've hardened to it by now. There's such an extraordinary turnover of junior doctors that I understand why there's no great fanfare. As a particularly venomous matron once hissed at us, 'You are temporary visitors at my permanent place of work.'

I've never once had a goodbye card, let alone a present. Until today, when I found a package in my pigeonhole from Mr Lockhart. A card to say thank you and goodbye, and a brand new Montblanc pen.

7

Registrar – Post Three

Eventually there comes a point where you have to decide what kind of doctor to be. Not the technical stuff, like whether you're into urology or neurology, but the more important matter of your bedside manner. Your stage persona evolves throughout your training but you generally settle on a way of dealing with patients a couple of years in, and carry it through into your consultant career. Are you smiley, charming and positive? Quiet, contemplative and scientific? I presume it's the same decision policemen make when they decide if they're good cop or bad cop (or racist cop).

I went for a 'straight to the point' vibe – no nonsense, no small talk, let's deal with the matter in hand, a bit of sarcasm thrown into the mix. Two reasons, really. It was already my personality, so there wasn't too much acting involved, plus it saves an awful lot of your day if you don't do the five-minute preamble about the weather, their job and their journey every fucking time. It sets you up as a bit distant but I don't think that's such a bad thing; I didn't really want patients trying to add me on

Facebook or asking what colour they should paint their downstairs bog.

The conventional teaching is that patients want doctors to ask open questions ('Tell me about your concerns . . .'), then give them a variety of treatment options, from conservative to medical to surgical, so the patient can make their own decisions. Terms like 'choice' sound good in theory – we all like to feel we are masters of our own destinies – but have you ever been in a canteen queue where there are more than a couple of mains? People dither, they change their minds, they look for affirmation from friends. Is the haddock nice? How about the shepherd's pie? I don't really know what I fancy. And all the while, your chips are getting cold. Sometimes, it's best to cut to the chase and remove any room for doubt.

On labour ward especially, I found that patients gained confidence from their doctors advocating a single management plan – you need the patient to be calm and trust you implicitly with their life and the life of their baby. Likewise, in clinic I saved countless patients delays to effective treatment by not proffering a specials board of options that are almost certainly of no benefit, just so I can say there's been patient choice. Instead I've offered my expert opinion; the patient's choice is whether or not to take it. It's what I'd personally want if I saw a doctor myself, or even if I took my car to the garage.

But there's no hiding from the fact that a direct approach makes you a less 'nice' doctor. Being trusted is much more important than being liked, but it's good to have the whole set, so I decided in my third post as a registrar – now working in a huge teaching hospital – to warm up my bedside manner. It wasn't totally spontaneous, I'll admit; someone had complained about me. It was about my clinical performance rather than my behaviour, but it so totally floored me that I realized I needed to do everything in my power to never attract a complaint again, and if that involved hairdresser-style chit-chat and an elbow-to-elbow smile then so be it.

A letter arrived at home out of the blue from the hospital I'd worked at two years previously, letting me know a patient I had operated on was suing me for medical negligence. As it happens, I wasn't negligent – bladder injury occurs in 1:200 caesareans, and she was informed of this risk pre-operatively on the consent form she signed. I'd like to think the risk of *me* injuring your bladder is considerably less than 1:200, as I only did it once and had many more than 200 other opportunities to do so. I felt terrible at the time it happened, but knew it had been managed well – I spotted what I'd done immediately, the urologists came to repair it straight away, and although it must have been distressing for the patient, ultimately it resulted in nothing more than a slightly delayed discharge home. I also thought it was managed well with her afterwards: I was apologetic, honest and humble, which in this case didn't require any acting at all. The last thing you want to do to a patient is actually give them one of the complications you warn them about. First, do no harm; it's right at the top of the job description. But, shit happens, and on that occasion it happened to her.

Messrs Cunt, Cuntsome and Cuntiest – solicitors of the ambulance-pursuing 'no win, no fee' persuasion – took a different view. According to their expert opinion, which seemed to have been honed from skim-reading a book called *Law: Just Throw the Fucking Lot at Them and See Who Gets Back Up Again*, the trust was negligent, I carried out the operation well below the standard reasonably expected of me, I greatly extended the suffering of the claimant and I delayed her opportunity to bond with her newborn child.

Unfortunately, I wasn't able to counter sue for the hours needlessly spent going through old medical records, taking meetings with lawyers and defence unions or the damage inflicted on my relationship by eroding the precious little time we spent together, nor the cost of the Red Bulls that kept me awake on night shifts after sleepless days of report-writing. Or the suffering *I* felt – the anxiety and guilt mounted onto an already stressful working life, the unfairness of being accused of being terrible at my job, the fear that maybe I *was* terrible at my job. I always tried my absolute hardest for every patient I saw and it was like a dagger through my heart for anyone to suggest otherwise.

The patient almost certainly had no idea how sad and exhausting the process would be for me – her lawyer no doubt smoothed down his moustache, put on his best concerned face and told her it was worth a roll of the dice in case it resulted in a nice payout* – and he was right, the hospital settled out of court, as they generally do. Maybe it's just part of the gradual Americanization of the health service, that it necessarily becomes more litigious. Or maybe the patient was one of those joyless types who sues half the people she meets: the bus driver who doesn't say good morning; the waiter who forgets her side of fries; me again for writing about all this. Whatever was going on behind the scenes, it left me at my lowest ebb as a registrar – asking myself why I bothered in the first place if now even the patients had it in for me. I seriously considered jacking it all in, something that had never occurred to me before. But I didn't. I decided I would scrabble desperately around for a positive to take from it, which was to do my very best to protect myself from any future letters on legal headed notepaper.

'Good morning!' beamed Adam 2.0 in a typically over-running antenatal clinic.

'You taking the piss, mate?' said the patient's husband. And so my revamp lasted two days.

---

* It would never be the doctor ending up personally out of pocket in a situation like this. The hospital will foot the bill, or a medical defence organization in the case of GPs. There can sometimes be a criminal case too if it's considered gross negligence – and a complaint to the GMC can run in tandem with any legal complaint, jeopardizing your registration and ability to practise.

Friday, 6 February 2009

Patient HJ needs an emergency caesarean section for failure to progress in labour. This has not come as a surprise. When I met her on admission, she presented me with her nine-page birth plan, in full colour and laminated. The whale song that would be playing on her laptop (I don't recall the exact age and breed of the whale, but I'm pretty sure it was documented to that level of detail), the aromatherapy oils that would be used, an introduction to the hypnotherapy techniques she would be employing, a request for the midwife to say 'surges' rather than 'contractions'. The whole thing was doomed from the start – having a birth plan always strikes me as akin to having a 'what I want the weather to be' plan or a 'winning the lottery' plan. Two centuries of obstetricians have found no way of predicting the course of a labour, but a certain denomination of floaty-dressed mother seems to think she can manage it easily.

Needless to say, HJ's birth plan has gone right up the fuck. Hypnotherapy has given way to gas and air has given way to an epidural. The midwife tells me the patient snapped at her husband to 'turn that bullshit off' when he was fiddling with the volume on the whale grunts. She's been stuck at 5 cm dilatation for the best part of six hours despite Syntocinon.* We've 'given it a couple more hours' twice now, so I explain baby isn't going to come out vaginally and I'm not prepared to wait until it inevitably becomes distressed and there's a huge emergency. We're going to need to perform a caesarean section. As expected, this doesn't go down particularly well. 'Come on!' she says. 'There must be a third way!'

I'm loath to court a PALS† complaint from a patient who wants their birth to be blogpost-perfect and has somehow been let down by nature. I've had a complaint in the past from a patient who I refused to allow to have candles burning while she laboured. 'I don't think it's such an unreasonable request,' she wrote. About having naked flames right next to oxygen tanks.

This patient's got 'strongly worded email' written all over her, so I cover myself by asking the consultant to pop by and have a quick chat with her. Luckily, Mr Cadogan is on duty – he's fatherly, charming and soothing, and he smells expensive, which has posh women

---

* Syntocinon (synthetic oxytocin) is an intravenous drug that increases contractions and speeds up a labour. You're meant to progress by a centimetre of dilatation every hour or two, and if that's not happening despite Syntocinon then it's caesarean time.

† PALS (Patient Advice and Liaison Services) are the hospital's complaints department. They take 'the customer is always right' to bizarre new heights and no matter how trivial the complaint would gladly have doctors turn up at patients' houses carrying a bouquet of flowers and wearing a hair shirt.

flocking to the private ward he'd much rather be on. He soon has HJ consented for theatre. He even offers to do the section himself, to quiet mutterings of derision and amazement from the other staff. No one here can remember the last time he delivered a baby for free. Perhaps golf's been rained off?

He suggests to the patient that he performs something called a 'natural caesarean' – it's the first time I've heard of such a thing. The theatre lights are dimmed, classical music plays and baby is allowed to slowly emerge from the tummy while both parents watch. It's a gimmick, and no doubt attracts a huge premium as part of his Platinum Package or whatever, but HJ laps it up. It's the first time she's looked remotely happy all day. With Mr Cadogan out of the room, HJ asks the midwife what she thinks about 'natural caesareans'. 'If that guy was operating on *me*,' the midwife replies, 'I'd want the lights turned up as high as they go.'

Saturday, 7 February 2009

Missed the first half of *Les Mis* thanks to a tricky caesarean at twenty-nine weeks,* and didn't have the

---

* Caesarean sections are much more difficult for premature babies. The lower segment, which you normally cut through at full term, doesn't properly form until around thirty-two weeks. This means you have to go through a much thicker part of the uterus, making it a harder and bloodier procedure.

fuckingest clue what was going on in the second half. (Especially as the goodie, Jean Valjean, and the baddie, Javert, essentially have the same name.)

Debriefing with Ron and the others in the pub afterwards, watching the first half didn't seem to have helped anyone else understand it either.

Sunday, 8 February 2009

Simon called to say he'd cut his wrists last night after a fight with his new girlfriend and ended up in hospital for a bunch of stitches. He's back home now and doing OK, with psychiatry follow-up arranged.

He asked if I was angry with him and I said of course I wasn't. I was actually extremely angry – that he'd done it, that he hadn't called me first so I could attempt to talk him down; surely he owed me that after the hours of time I've given him? I felt guilty that I hadn't done enough – that I should have helped him better, or seen it coming and stopped it. And then I felt guilty about being so angry with him.

We chatted for an hour or so and I reminded him he can call me any time, day or night. But we've had this chat so often in the last three years, and it's miserable to think that we're no further forward than when he posted that first cry for help.

Actually, that's probably the wrong way of looking at it. You don't cure depression, the same way you don't cure asthma; you manage it. I'm the inhaler he's decided to go with and I should be pleased he's gone this long without an attack.

Tuesday, 17 February 2009

The emergency buzzer goes and it's a slightly tricky situation to restore calm in. As well as the usual dozen people buzzing around, there's dust and rubble everywhere, and panic as a result. If this were an episode of *Casualty*, there'd be half an ambulance smashed into the room with us, but no. The midwife has pulled the emergency cord so hard she's taken down most of the ceiling.

Thursday, 19 February 2009

It's a great shame our child protection duties[*] don't extend to vetoing some of the terrible names parents saddle their unfortunate babies with. This morning I delivered little baby Sayton – pronounced Satan, as in King of the Underworld. It's hard to believe he'll get through his school career unbullied, and yet we merrily wave him off on that journey. (Or maybe he's actually the devil and I should have just shoved him back in.)

At lunch, fierce discussion with my colleague Katie as to whether my run-in with baby Sayton is better or

---

[*] All doctors have a duty, enshrined in their GMC code, to protect children and young people from abuse and neglect by acting on any concerns they have.

worse than one she delivered called LeSanya, pronounced Lasagne, as in Lasagne. We regularly compare horror stories, like we're playing Top Trumps: Obstetrics.

She tells me she once pulled out a baby girl called Clive, though I point out we've got a Princess Michael, so that's not particularly impressive. Oliver says that where he was born, in Iceland, names must be picked from a specific list, from which it's illegal to deviate. Doesn't sound like the worst idea.

Wednesday, 4 March 2009

It shouldn't be a notable event when I manage to leave labour ward on time, but today I do, and have a long-arranged dinner with Grandma in Teddington. She leans over after starters, licks her finger and wipes a dot of food off my cheek. As she licks her finger again, I realize slightly too late that it was a patient's vaginal blood. I decide not to mention it.

Saturday, 7 March 2009

'Doctor Adam! You delivered my baby!' squeals the woman behind the cheese counter at Sainsbury's. I have no recollection of her whatsoever, but her story seems to check out – that is, after all, my name and occupation. I ask about 'the little one', as obviously I have no memory of the baby's gender. He's doing well. She asks me ridiculously specific questions relating to the vagina-side small talk I had with her a year ago: how I got on with building the shed, if Costco stayed open until 8 p.m. on Thursdays like I'd hoped. I feel slightly guilty about the colossal mismatch in impressions we made on each other. But then again, I guess it was one of the most important moments of her life, and for me she may well have been delivery number six that day. It's a peek into what it must be like to be a celebrity, a fan asking you if you remember a meet-and-greet after a concert ten years ago.

'I'll put it through as Cheddar,' she whispers to me as she weighs my goat's cheese – it'll save me a couple of quid and will therefore be one of the biggest perks of the job I've ever had. I smile at her.

'That's not Cheddar, Rose,' announces her supervisor as he stalks past, and my bonus evaporates.

Monday, 30 March 2009

I've just printed off a scan of their baby for some parents and am wiping the ultrasound jelly off mum, when dad asks if I can take another picture from a different angle, saying, 'I'm just not sure I can put this one up on Facebook.' My eyebrows are en route to my hairline at these life-chronicling, self-obsessed social media attention-seekers when I take a closer look at the photo. I see what he means: it very much appears that the fetus is wanking.

Friday, 3 April 2009

Having a drink with Ron – we're talking about his job and how he's decided it's 'time to move on'. I sometimes think about the idea of moving on myself, but it's a slightly alien concept when I only have one possible employer in the country. He offers to set me up with his recruitment consultant and tells me he's sure I've got plenty of transferable skills.

I hear this a lot from non-medics, but I don't really buy it. The feeling is that doctors are expert problem-solvers, who pull together a constellation of symptoms to deduce a unique diagnosis. The reality is we're more Dr Nick than Dr House. We learn to recognize a limited set of specific problems from patterns we've seen before – like a two-year-old who can point and say 'cat' and 'duck', but would struggle to identify a breeze block or a chaise longue. I strongly suspect I wouldn't last long as a management consultant, applying my problem-solving skills to a failing branch of La Senza.

'You should absolutely be on six figures by now,' says Ron, texting me the contact details of his recruiter. I tell him I'll get in touch with her, but I'm not sure I want to. I'm not convinced she'll want *me* either when I outline my core competency: pulling babies and Kinder Eggs out of vaginas.

Monday, 6 April 2009

Eyes down for an elective caesarean section – this time for placenta praevia.[*] In the event, a very straight-forward one, but everyone is quiet and focused in case it gets messy. Everyone, that is, except the dad, who is determined to engage me in pitiful banter.

'Whoa, I'm glad she's got skin covering that the rest of the time', 'This must put you off women, doc', something about the baby's penis and the umbilical cord – all the classics. I presume it's just because he's nervous, but it's extremely irritating and distracting, and none of his lines would even make it onto the speech bubble of a saucy seaside postcard. I 'mm-hm' at his zingers, and all but say, 'I'm really trying to concentrate here. Let me deliver this baby. I didn't rock up at the conception and distract you from your pumping with my pound-shop repartee.'

He continues. 'Better not come out black, eh? Ever had a baby come out a different colour to the parents?'

'Does blue count?' I offer. Banter over.

---

[*] Placenta praevia is a placenta that is attached at the lower part of the uterus. The implications of this are that the baby needs to be delivered by caesarean because the placenta's in the way for deliver-ing vaginally. It also means that if mum goes into labour, it's a bit of an emergency as the placenta is liable to shear off, with profound consequences for both baby and mother (700 ml of blood goes through the placenta every minute – her entire blood volume in five minutes).

Patient JS is twenty-two years old and has presented to A&E with acute abdominal pain. The A&E officer tells me she's had a negative pregnancy test and has been reviewed by the surgeons, who suspect it's probably a gynae issue. I review her. She looks reasonably well – pulse a bit high, tummy a bit tender, but walking and talking easily. Admitting her to the ward would be over-kill, and sending her home would probably be underkill. If this was a daytime shift during the week I'd probably just squeeze her onto someone's ultrasound list to check there's nothing sinister going on. But it's a Saturday night and the NHS runs a skeleton service. Actually, that's unfair on skeletons – it's more like when they dig up remains of Neolithic Man and reconstruct what he might have looked like from a piece of clavicle and a thumb joint.

One would generally err on the side of caution and admit her until she can be scanned in the morning, wasting a night of the patient's life rather than sacrific-ing my career if I've called it wrong. It also wastes the cost of a hospital bed, which is around the £400 mark. I suspect the cost of an ultrasonography shift would be considerably lower than this, and you'd save at least one such admission a night, but who am I to tell the hospital how to spend their money? Particularly when they've just decided to get rid of the beds from our on-call rooms. (Perhaps they'll save money on the bed linen they remember to change every week or two? Perhaps they were worried morale was running a little too high? That doctors would be too alert, too on it, if they got some sleep?)

We're OK in obs and gynae – the Early Pregnancy Assessment Unit sister took pity on us, no doubt clocking the size of the bags under our eyes, and had a spare key cut so we can kip on a hospital bed in her unit. It's an act of charity so kind and so rare that it made my colleague Fleur cry, and then scour the honours website trying to work out if Sister would be eligible for an OBE. It's hard to describe the joy of hearing you'll have a bed to lie in, after a few night shifts spent trying to snatch some sleep in an office chair. It's a bed with stirrups, but beggars can't be choosers; I'd have accepted a bed with a grand piano dangling from the ceiling above it by a single pube if there was any chance of some shut-eye.

I suddenly realize it's also a bed with an ultrasound machine sat next to it. I check JS is still good to walk, and take her off upstairs – if all looks well on a quick scan she can head home, and I won't even bill the NHS the £400 I've saved them through my ingenuity.

In retrospect, it was a mistake to not tell the A&E sister I was borrowing the patient. I imagined being informed of some bit of protocol that meant I wouldn't be allowed to, and nobody's got time for that kind of argument. It was also a mistake not to book a porter to take her up with me in a wheelchair. But the biggest mistake of all was definitely made by the A&E officer who told me the patient had had a negative pregnancy test – unless 'negative pregnancy test' is the rather confusing term he uses for 'I have not performed a pregnancy test'.

By the time we've gone upstairs, through a depressing lab-rat maze of corridors and into my makeshift bedroom with en-suite ultrasound machine, JS is looking a little peaky and a lot out of breath. Ultrasound of her abdomen shows a ruptured ectopic pregnancy, her belly swimming with blood. Instead of being where she should be, in close proximity to life-saving equipment, she's kicking back with me in a closed-off part of the hospital, like we're two teenagers who've slunk off for a snog.

Half an hour of panicked phone calls later, we're in theatre, JS is a few bags of blood better off, a fallopian tube worse off, and will be absolutely fine. I have no idea what the moral of this story is.

Sunday, 26 April 2009

Called to review a patient in A&E. According to her notes she is aged thirty-five and employed in a massage parlour, in a capacity one suspects doesn't involve a whole lot of massaging – at least not with her hands. She presents with a lost object in her vagina. A busy shift, so no time for too many questions, and it's legs up, lights on, speculum in, see it, grab it, remove it. Without doubt, this is the worst smell I've ever experienced. Truly indescribable – other than to say that I retch, and the nurse chaperone has to immediately leave the cubicle. I imagine every bunch of flowers in the hospital suddenly wilted. I hardly want to ask, but I need to know the culprit.

The short answer is it was the head of a Fireman Sam bath sponge. But of course! The long answer is she realized a number of months ago her income was being seriously compromised because there were certain dates of the month when her clients didn't want to be 'massaged' – so she created an impromptu menstrual barrier device by decapitating Samuel. Christ knows how she explained the change in his appearance to her children – did any of them notice? Were they worried they'd be for the guillotine next if they asked as to its whereabouts? While effective at soaking up menstrual blood from above, and quite noticeably effective at absorbing other fluids from below, Sam's bonce-barrier didn't have a string to facilitate its removal. Plus it had been schnitzeled flat by her clients' pummellings over the past three months.

Actually, it's unfair to say the smell was indescribable – it's describable as three months of menstrual blood mixed with vaginal secretions and the fetid semen of assorted men, the number of whom must have run into three figures. While prescribing her some antibiotics, I let her know that no further novelty sponges needed to be executed in her honour – she can also stop her periods by the more traditional method of taking the oral contraceptive pill back to back. I leave it to A&E to decide how to label the item within the microbiology sample pot.

Monday, 4 May 2009

Another day, another emergency buzzer or twelve. I go to perform a ventouse extraction for a non-reassuring trace, but as I'm about to Dyson the little bastard out of there the trace improves so I take my gloves off and hand back over to the midwife for a normal delivery. I loiter at the back of the room to keep an eye on the trace in case it misbehaves again, but all is well and soon baby's head is crowning.

Dad is down the business end, witnessing the miracle of childbirth for the first time – awwing, cooing and excitedly telling his wife how brilliantly she's doing. The midwife tells mum to stop pushing and start panting, so she can guide baby's head out slowly and hopefully avoid too much of a tear. As the head advances, dad screams, 'Oh my God – where's its face?!' Mum understandably also screams, her baby's head shoots out uncontrolled and her perineum explodes. I explain to them that babies are generally born facing downwards,*

---

* Only 5 per cent of babies are born looking upwards – the medical term for which is 'occipito-posterior'. The cutesy-wutesy term is 'star-gazing', the old-fashioned term is 'face to pubis', and the term

and their baby's face looks perfect (if slightly more blood-splattered than it might have been). I put some gloves on and open a suture set.

Tuesday, 5 May 2009

Patient in antenatal clinic requests a caesarean section without a clinical indication. I explain our unit doesn't perform caesareans on request: there needs to be a medical reason, because it's an operation, with attendant risks of bleeding, infection, anaesthetic and so on. Her argument was she didn't want to go through a long labour and then end up with an emergency caesarean. I was obviously bang to rights – a planned section is much safer than an emergency one, and generally safer than an instrumental delivery too – but couldn't say so.

She wasn't done trying. 'Aabaat fimetoo poshtapush?' she said in her finest estuary drawl, which I eventually decoded as 'How about if I'm too posh to push?' I felt mean saying no, especially as a third of female obstetricians elect for caesareans – it's clearly not fair.

I was on the other side of the fence yesterday. H and I were looking to upsize mildly and were going round a flat we liked with an estate agent. The barely twenty-year-old weasel was doing the hard sell; it's a great location, we were told – he bought his own place on the

---

I misheard as a junior SHO and then mortifyingly used for a year, until I was corrected by a colleague, is 'face to pubes'.

road behind. This made it all the more depressing; an embryo in shiny nylon could spare the cash to buy a flat somewhere we can barely afford. Was I in the wrong job? Or is an estate agency like a charity shop, where the staff get first dibs on everything that comes in?

He told us the sellers of this place had previously rejected a below-asking-price offer, but he couldn't tell me how far below asking price – it's against estate agents' weasel-law, a code of honour among the dishonourable. I asked him if his colleagues tipped him the wink about how far below asking price any other offers were when he was buying his own flat. He went a delightful shade of sun-dried tomato. 'Ask me my favourite number of pounds!' he said. Turns out his favourite number was 11,500.

'Ask me why some women have caesareans,' I said to the patient. I waited for her intellectual satellite delay to catch up, and she asked. I answered that some women are worried about the significantly worse long-term effects of normal deliveries on bladder and bowel continence, as it would markedly affect their lifestyle. Turns out she was too, and is now booked in for an elective caesarean at thirty-nine weeks.

Thursday, 25 June 2009

Down in A&E around 11 p.m. to review a patient, and thumbing through Twitter while I work up the strength to see her. There's a big news story breaking, but so far only gossip-merchants TMZ have reported it. 'Oh Christ,' I gasp. 'Michael Jackson's dead!' One of the nurses sighs and stands up. 'Which cubicle?'

Saturday, 18 July 2009

If they're updating the Hippocratic oath any time soon, they should add in a line about never mentioning you're a doctor at parties. Particularly for obs and gynae staff, where it opens up an entire hell-mouth of discussion with every woman on the planet – questions about contraception or fertility or pregnancy. I've become extremely good at being vague about what I do when I meet new people, or magically changing the subject.

At a house party tonight, conversation turns to the niqab, and someone chips in that underneath their niqabs a lot of women wear very high-end fashion, often thousands of pounds of clothing hidden from view. 'It's true,' I say. 'And underneath *that* I've seen so many orthodox Muslim women with Agent Provocateur lingerie, and half a dozen with really elaborate pubic topiary. Initials shaved in, spirals, the lot!' Absolute silence. Then I realize that I've overdone it on the mystery. 'I'm a doctor by the way.'

Tuesday, 28 July 2009

Booking a couple in for an elective caesarean and they ask me if there's any chance they could choose a particular date. They're a British Chinese couple, and I know that according to the Chinese zodiac, certain days of the year are lucky or unlucky, and it's of course preferable to deliver on an 'auspicious date', as it's known.

Obviously we'll try our best to accommodate this, if safe and practicable. They ask me to check for the first or second of September. 'Auspicious dates?' I ask, smiling and mentally clearing a space on my lapel for an 'excellence in cultural sensitivity' badge.

'No,' the husband replies. 'September babies go into a different school year and perform better in exams.'

Monday, 10 August 2009

Yes, madam, you *will* shit during labour. Yes, it's completely normal. It's a pressure thing. No, there's nothing I can do to stop it. Although if you'd asked me yesterday I'd have suggested that the massive curry you ate to 'induce labour'* probably wasn't going to help matters.

Monday, 17 August 2009

Teaching the medical students a bit of pelvic anatomy when someone from med school administration appears

---

* Curry can't induce labour. Nor can pineapple. Nor can sex. There is no scientific evidence whatsoever for these three perennial old wives' tales. I presume they were dreamt up by the inventor of the pineapple madras when he was horny.

with news of Justin, the missing member of the group. He won't be joining us for the rest of the term, and it sounds very much like he won't be joining the medical profession at all. Last night, he got into a fist fight with his boyfriend at a nightclub and the police were called. The police spotted that Justin had a quantity of white powder on him; they suspected it wasn't Canderel and arrested him on the spot. Justin's defence was that he should be immediately released on the basis that he's a medical student and his country needs him. This back-fired ever so slightly and the police contacted the medical school, accounting for his absence this morning.

The administrator leaves and no one's particularly interested in learning pelvic anatomy any more (if they ever were). We have a discussion about fitness to prac-tise among medical students and getting struck off before you even get struck on. Every single student asks at least one gossamer thinly veiled 'What if a student did *this*?' hypothetical question, before each of their faces drains of colour on hearing my answer. I regale them with the story of some contemporaries of mine who got sent down. A bunch of third years were on a rugby tour in France; a tour that consisted of the odd game of rugby and countless hours of drinking games. The most inventive of these games involved visiting local hostelries and making 'Very Bloody Marys'. They would order large measures of vodka from the bar, return to their tables, produce needles and syringes, venesect each other, squirt blood into each other's vodkas and then neck them. The gendarmerie point-blank ignored the rule of 'what goes on tour stays on tour' and responded quite urgently to the bar staff's concerns about all the discarded needles on their premises, arresting the students and informing the university. My tutorial group seemed happy that this was a striking-off offence, although one raised the mitigating factor that it's pretty impressive for a group of third years to be able to take blood.

'Poor Justin' still seemed to be the prevailing feeling amongst them. My suggested 'Poor Justin's beaten-up boyfriend' fell on fairly deaf ears.

'I just can't believe it,' one girl sighed loudly. 'Justin's *gay?*'

Wednesday, 19 August 2009

Moral maze. Working my way through the day's elective caesareans. This one is for breech presentation – I·cut through the uterus and the baby quite clearly isn't breech. Fuck. I should have scanned the baby before I started – you're always meant to, just in case the baby has turned since the last ultrasound. Which it never has. Except today.

My choices are as follows:

a) Deliver the magical revolving baby and confess to the patient I've done a completely unnecessary caesarean section, scarred her abdomen and confined her to hospital for a few days, when she could have had a normal delivery.

b) Deliver the baby and pretend it was breech – this would involve lying in the notes, and persuading my assistant and scrub nurse to perjure themselves by colluding.

c) Stick my hand inside the uterus, rotate the baby, grab a leg and deliver it breech.

I choose a) and fess up to the remarkably understanding patient, who I suspect actually wanted a caesarean in any case. Then it's time to fill in the clinical incident form and tell Mr Cadogan. He's very nice about it and says at least I'll never forget to scan a patient before a section again.

He also makes me feel much better by telling me about an unnecessary section he once performed as a junior trainee. Baby wasn't coming out with forceps, so he performed an emergency caesarean. Unfortunately, when he got inside the abdomen, the baby had somehow delivered vaginally in the meantime.

'How did you explain *that* to the patient?!' I ask.

There's a pause. 'Well, we weren't always quite so honest with the punters back then.'

Thursday, 20 August 2009

I consent patient YS for Termination of Pregnancy – an unplanned, unwanted pregnancy in a twenty-year-old student following condom failure. We discuss alternative

methods of contraception and correct condom usage.[*]
I identify an error in her technique. I'm as big a fan of
recycling as the next man, but if you turn a used condom
inside out and put it back on for round two, it's probably not going to be that effective.[†]

Tuesday, 20 October 2009

We're one registrar down in antenatal clinic, so I'm
sailing this shitshow alone. I saw thirty patients in

---

[*] I performed a large number of TOPs in this job, as a lot of the other
junior doctors had objections for ethical or religious reasons (or pre-
tended to, because they're work-shy bastards). No one's first choice
of a way to spend a morning, but a necessary evil, and as a result I
developed excellent surgical technique for ERPC – the near-identical
surgical procedure required following certain miscarriages. By now
I could probably hoover the stairs through my letter box if needed.
This patient didn't want to raise a child, and we live in a civilized
society – it's not fair on her or the child to force her to go through
with it, a fact that, depressingly, it took Ireland until 2018 to realize
and, even more depressingly, Northern Ireland still doesn't acknowledge. According to the letter of the law (the 1967 Abortion Act to be
precise), two doctors need to agree that continuing with a pregnancy
would be damaging to the patient's mental health, but in reality that
covers any unwanted pregnancy. In this case the patient had
attempted to take reasonable precautions against falling pregnant.
Used correctly, condoms can be 98 per cent effective, but frequent
mistakes include late application, early removal and incorrect lubrication, so it's always good to check they're being used properly.

[†] A couple of years later, I encountered an example of condom failure where the guy thought that because a condom was coated with
spermicide, and he didn't really like the feeling of them, he could roll
it on to coat his cock with spermicide, then take it off before sex.

morning clinic, which finished at 3 p.m., two hours after my afternoon clinic was meant to have started.

All the patients I see are pissed off, and rightly so – they've been sitting in a waiting room for four hours, crotchety as a pen of wet hens. Safe to say my sincere apologies and not-my-faults don't count for much while they grunt their way through their appointments. I strongly suspect if I was a pilot and my co-pilot didn't turn up, the airline might find a better solution than 'plough ahead and see what happens'.

Seven p.m. and two patients from the finish line I have to make an urgent psychiatric referral for someone who's had a relapse of severe anorexia nervosa at thirty weeks. And she's eaten more than I have today.

Wednesday, 28 October 2009

I need to admit a woman for pelvic inflammatory disease, to receive intravenous antibiotics. Unfortunately, she doesn't want to receive any because she thinks I'm in the pocket of the pharmaceutical industry, so we've reached a bit of a stalemate. We talk through her concerns. It turns out this is a very recent worry, having read something about it on Facebook yesterday.

Yet another mark against technology as far as I'm concerned. The trust have finally acknowledged we're in the twenty-first century and digitized our radiology system, doing away with all light boxes and physical printed X-rays. Instead we can now access them from any computer in the hospital. Unfortunately, the system has been broken since they installed it, thereby putting our practice back to the nineteenth century, before the introduction of X-rays.

Patients frequently attend clinic with reams of paper they've googled, printed off and highlighted, and it's pretty tedious spending an extra ten minutes per patient explaining why a blogger in Copenhagen who uses a pink hearts Wordpress theme might not be a reliable source. Then again, if it wasn't for Google I wouldn't be able to send patients off for a urine sample while I look things up in a panic.

Today technology is serving up conspiracy theories. The patient asks me to prove I'm not being bribed by drug companies. I point out that the antibiotics I want to put her on cost a matter of pennies, and that drug companies would probably be furious with me for not choosing something more expensive. She doesn't waver. I point out that the antibiotics I've prescribed are generic[*] rather than pushing one company's product. Still unmoved. I point out that I drive a five-year-old Peugeot 206, so I'm probably as far out of anyone's pocket as is possible. 'Fine,' she says and agrees to the antibiotics.

---

[*] Almost any drug you get at the chemist comes in both branded and cheaper generic forms. Panadol is a brand name for the generic drug paracetamol, Amoxil is a brand name for amoxicillin.

Wednesday, 4 November 2009

Patient TH is an accountant in her mid-thirties, who has been diagnosed with an ectopic pregnancy. She is a candidate for medical management using methotrexate,* and is keen to do so and avoid surgery. I consent her for receiving the drug, and talk through the follow-up procedure. I explain the possible side effects and the various 'dos and don'ts' while on treatment, emphasizing that she must use effective contraception for the next three months and abstain from sex altogether for the first month after treatment. She pauses to consider this, before asking, 'How about anal?'†

Wednesday, 18 November 2009

Visiting Ron's dad in hospital. He looks terrible, jaundiced skin stretched tight over jutting bone. A roadmap of blood vessels is visible across his face where his body has burnt away every single fat cell, throwing all its energy at fighting a cancer it has no chance against. 'I wish people didn't have to see me like this,' he says.

---

* Certain patients with ectopic pregnancies can be managed with a drug called methotrexate, if they're medically well and the ectopic is small. It's a pretty nuclear drug which attacks rapidly dividing cells, meaning it's effective at dissolving the ectopic pregnancy and can also be used in chemotherapy.

† If you're interested, the answer is 'yes, even anal'. There's still a risk of the ectopic pregnancy rupturing, so we try to avoid any prangs in that neck of the woods.

'We'll be spending a fortune on the undertakers making me look nice afterwards – can't you just wait a few more months?'

He's in hospital for an oesophageal stent insertion so he can continue to eat and drink, to make his final chapter as comfortable as possible. The retired engineer in him is fascinated by the mechanism of the stent, a self-expanding metallic mesh, strong enough to push back the tumour and open up his gullet. 'Wouldn't have been possible twenty years ago,' he says, and we talk about being lucky to live in this current blink of civilization's eye. 'Do you think they'll be able to cure cancer twenty years from now?' he asks. I can't work out whether saying yes or no would be more comforting. I deflect with, 'I only know about vaginas, pal,' and he laughs.

Next question. 'Why do we always say that people lost their battle with cancer, and never that cancer won its battle against them?' He keeps making jokes – to be fair, he's done it the entire time I've known him. I find it uncomfortable for the first few minutes of my visit, but I'm soon genuinely enjoying a morning I'd been dreading. It's a kind and clever move – it doesn't just make it easier for his friends and family when they visit, it also means we'll remember him as he always was, diminished physically maybe, but not in personality.

Thursday, 10 December 2009

A poignant ventouse delivery – it's a mum I saw in infertility clinic at the start of this job. I feel like holding the baby aloft like Simba and blasting out my best 'Circle of Life'.

While I'm patching her up, I ask how her fertility treatment went – turns out she got pregnant without any treatment the week after our appointment. Still, I'm taking it.

Thursday, 17 December 2009

Tragically, domestic abuse in pregnancy is still responsible for the deaths of mothers and babies every year in this country. Every obstetrician has a duty to look out for it. This is often difficult as controlling husbands are likely to attend clinics with their wives, denying them an opportunity to speak up. Our hospital has a system to help women disclose abuse – in the ladies' toilet there is a sign that says 'If you want to discuss any concerns about violence at home, put a red sticker on the front of your notes', and there are sheets of red-dot stickers in every cubicle.

Today, for the first time in my career, a woman has dotted a few red stickers on the front of her notes. It's a tricky situation as she's attended clinic with her husband and two-year-old child. I try and fail to get the husband to leave the room. I call in the senior midwife and consultant and between us we get her alone.

As gently as we interrogate, it's not doing any good; she's clamming up – scared, confused. After ten minutes we establish that the red dots were the early artistic efforts of her two-year-old, who stuck them on the notes when they went to the toilet together.

8

Registrar – Post Four

During my career as a doctor, for every 'would you mind having a look at this lump/rash/penis?' I heard off-duty, there was always one 'I don't know how you do it'. I generally heard it from people who wouldn't qualify for jury service, let alone from medical school, but it's still a valid point. It's a difficult job in terms of hours, energy and emotion; and from the outside a pretty unenviable one.

By the time I was six years deep into medicine, the shine had definitely rubbed off the surface. On more than one occasion my finger had hovered over the 'fuck it' button – days where things had gone wrong, patients had complained, rotas had changed at the last minute – and my resolve wavered. Not quite enough to start circling the jobs page of the paper, but certainly enough to wonder if I might have any long-lost millionaire aunts on their way out.

But there were two things keeping me there. Firstly, I'd worked long and hard to get as far as I had. Secondly – and I realize it might sound a bit worthy – it's a privilege to be allowed to play such an important role in people's lives.

You may be an hour late home, but you're an hour late home because you stopped a mother bleeding to death. You may have had forty women in an antenatal clinic designed for twenty, but that's forty women relying on you for the health of their babies. Even in the parts of the job you hate – for me it was urogynaecology clinic, a bunch of nans with pelvic floors like quicksand and their uteri stalagtite-ing into their thermals – each decision you make can immeasurably improve someone's quality of life. And then a patient sneezes, you have to get a mop and bucket, and you wish you'd plumped for a career in chartered accountancy.

You may curse the job and the hours, own voodoo effigies of the management and even carry a vial of ricin on you at all times in case you ever meet the health secretary, but on an individual basis you really care for all the patients.*

I must have been in this kind of upbeat mood in my fourth registrar posting when I accepted an invitation to represent medicine at my old school's careers fair. It involved a morning sitting behind a table, while a bunch of gangly fifth-formers lumbered around and asked me questions about my job. Or as it turned out, mostly asked a bunch of other people questions about their more interesting and better-paid jobs. My table definitely

---

* Except the ones who try and sue you.

looked the least appealing – everyone else had stacks of leaflets and bowls of pens, sweets and key rings. Deloitte were even handing out Krispy Kremes, which felt a bit like cheating. What should I have brought to entice people into a career in medicine? Toy stethoscopes? Amniotic fluid smoothies? Diaries with all your weekends, evenings and Christmases handily crossed out?

The students who did speak to me were clever, driven and erudite – I'm sure they would have all breezed into medical school if they chose to – and I found myself spending a lot of time discussing what's bad as well as good about the job. Even though I felt protective of my profession, particularly with the other tables around, Christ knows we need people to go into it with both eyes open. So I told them the truth: the hours are terrible, the pay is terrible, the conditions are terrible; you're underappreciated, unsupported, disrespected and frequently physically endangered. But there's no better job in the world.

Infertility clinic: helping couples to fall pregnant after years of trying, who've all but given up hope – it's difficult to explain how special that feels. It's something I'd happily do in my own time and for free (which is handy as I frequently did – those clinics overran by hours). Labour ward: a true rollercoaster, by which I mean everyone generally ends up alive and well despite the fact it seems to be against the very laws of nature. You dart from room to room, delivering any baby who gets sick or gets stuck, making an indelible mark on the lives of these patients. A low-grade superhero – your utility belt containing a scalpel, some tongs and a wipe-clean hoover.

The careers on the other tables had their obvious draws – the principal one being a shit-ton of cash every month – but there's no feeling like knowing you've saved a life. Not even that, half the time; just knowing you've made a difference is enough. You go home – however tired, late and blood-splattered – with a spring in your step that's hard to describe, feeling like you have a useful part to play in the world. I said this little speech about thirty times, and by the end of the morning I felt like I'd been through rigorous couples therapy – talking all the problems out, realizing the spark was still there after all.

I felt uplifted as I left the school hall, actively looking forward to hitting labour ward on Monday. What an honour it is to do this job – even if it is significantly worse than the sum of its parts. I stole a Deloitte dough-nut and headed home.*

And the next time someone asked me, 'Seriously, how do you do it?' I truly knew what the answer was. Although the reply I generally gave was, 'I like operating on strangers' vaginas,' which at least ended the conver-sation quickly.

---

* Full disclosure: I did also take a leaflet about their graduate entry scheme.

Friday, 5 February 2010

Doing an elective section for a woman who'd had three previous sections – her abdomen is absolutely rock-solid with adhesions. I call my senior registrar in to help, and demote the SHO to a spectator role. Scar tissue means that bowel is matted to bladder is matted to uterus is matted to muscle is matted to God-knows-what. It's like ten pairs of headphones have become tangled together, and then the whole thing has been encased in concrete.

The senior reg tells me it will take as long as it takes – we just need to be slow and methodical. Better that it takes three hours than the patient needs her bowel repaired and spends an extra week in hospital. We assume the pace of an arthritic archaeological dig. Every time it gets a bit easier and I speed up, the SR puts his hand on mine and I slow right down again.

Eventually there's nearly enough space to make the cut and deliver the baby – just one last loop of bowel to gently encourage away from the uterus. I'm in the process of peeling it off when the unmistakeable fetid stench of bowel contents fills the theatre. Shit. Literally. And we were so close.

The SR tells me to deliver the baby – he'll pop out

and bleep a bowel surgeon over to repair the damage.* My SHO interrupts sheepishly, 'Sorry, guys – that was *my* bowel . . .'

Saturday, 6 February 2010

I meet Euan, a friend from university halls, and his wife, Milly, for lunch in town – they're feeding me in return for picking my brains about fertility issues. The mains arrive and I switch from reminiscence mode to doctor mode. 'So. How long have you been trying then?'

'Seven months and two weeks,' replies Milly robotic-ally, like a cash machine dispensing a tenner. She's weirdly precise.

In fact, weird and precise would prove to be her watchwords, as she then dips into a tote bag to produce a folder, which she passes to me, stony-faced. I am clearly being granted sight of a document of colossal importance. I flick through page after page of spread-sheets; it takes me a moment to absorb the sheer horror of her magnum opus. This is a database of every time they've had sex since coming off contraception, along-side the dates of Milly's cycle and, distressingly, the length of the session and who was on top. Quite why this was documented in such detail I have no idea, unless

---

* To test for a bowel perforation, it's a remarkably similar method to locating a hole in the inner tube of a bike tyre. You fill the abdomen up with water and pump air through the patient's anus until you can see where the bubbles are coming from.

it was a deliberate attempt to suppress my appetite and keep the lunch bill down.

I'm totally distracted for the rest of the meal, unable to shake thoughts of my ex-flatmate's sexual positions and durations, and him clambering on and off, or out from under, with the regimented duty of a workhorse. I manage to collect myself long enough to give them some half-decent advice: giving up coffee and alcohol, the blood tests they should get from their GP, the point where they need referral to infertility clinic.

'Is it worth keeping the diary going?' asks Milly.

'Oh, definitely,' I say – partly so they don't think they've needlessly shown me a sex almanac and partly to give some poor infertility registrar a good giggle in a few months' time.

Tuesday, 9 February 2010

Today, as I was making a perineum look slightly more like a perineum after a forceps extraction, the midwife asks mum if she's happy for her baby to have a Vitamin K injection. The patient treats us to some tabloid newspaper sensationalist scare-story quackery – except it appears this woman may have been holding her paper upside down.

She declines the Vitamin K because 'vaccines give you arthritis'. The midwife patiently explains that Vitamin K isn't a vaccine, it's a vitamin, which is very important to help with baby's blood clotting. And it doesn't cause arthritis – maybe she's thinking of autism, which also isn't caused by vaccines. Which this injection isn't.

'Nah,' the mum says. 'I'm not taking any chances with my baby's health.'

Sunday, 14 February 2010

First Valentine's Day spent with H in four years. I suggest that, Valentine-wise, going out with a doctor is like having your birthday on the 29th of February.

A lovely Thai dinner at the Blue Elephant restaurant. At the end of the meal, the waiter brings over a pair of heart-shaped sweets in a beautifully carved wooden box. I eat mine whole. Turns out it was actually a candle.

Tuesday, 16 February 2010

Husband and wife are both in tears at the news that baby will need to come out of the sunroof for failure to progress in labour. The main sadness seems to be the husband's slightly odd obsession with being the first person to touch the baby. There isn't much time to muse upon why he might want to do this – perhaps he wants to break an enchanted spell or has superpowers he needs to transfer to his offspring – but he is really most insistent. Isn't there a way he can still be the person who touches her first? If he lifts her out at the end of the caesarean maybe?

He would definitely faint, vomit or both at what it looks like inside an abdomen: a casserole of flesh and giblets cooked up by someone irrevocably insane. Besides, it takes most trainees a good few sections before they can get a baby out by the head – unless he can quickly practise by scooping cantaloupe melons out of a swamp one-handed? Plus no one seems to realize there's a whole tricky ritual that takes time to learn, namely getting scrubbed and then into gown and gloves. Gloves! 'How about if we pass baby straight to you?' I suggest. 'We'll be wearing gloves so you'll be the first person to actually touch her.'

Sold.

Thursday, 25 February 2010

The emergency buzzer goes off in labour ward. The whole team runs down the corridor and none of us can see a room with a flashing light outside.

You'd think they might come up with a more high-tech system given lives are at stake, but we're stuck with the aeroplane passenger call set-up. One person presses a button, the entire place hears a piercing beep every couple of seconds, and then the cabin crew/obstetric team has to traipse up and down looking for a light, until they find whoever pressed it and can turn the noise off. If only I could swap medical emergencies for something as serene as refilling someone's G&T or a terrorist saying he's going to blow up the plane.

The alarm is still going and, with precious time draining away, we decide to go from room to room, checking in on every single labouring patient. Clearly one of the lights has broken.

No one seems to be having an emergency. Where else is there? Changing rooms, labour ward theatres, toilets, anaesthetic rooms, tea room – we split up like Scooby Doo and the gang to cover every inch of the ward. Nothing. A literal false alarm. Aside from the fact it's deafeningly loud, every single member of staff is conditioned to react to this sound by leaping into action. It's too unsettling for background noise, much like if the radio started playing an air-raid siren.

We call engineering. Some bloke comes up and fucks around uselessly with a box on the wall for ten minutes. They'll get someone over to fix it tomorrow, apparently – until then we have the choice of a constantly blaring alarm or no alarm system at all. We summon Prof. Carrow, the on-call consultant, and he's furious. Mostly because he's spent the last decade successfully avoiding walking onto labour ward during his shifts, and also – as he points out to the engineer – this counts as an extremely serious clinical incident. Lives are being endangered and the company needs to come out immediately to resolve it. The engineer mutters he'll do his best, but no promises – and besides, what happened on labour wards a hundred years ago, before emergency buzzers?

Prof. Carrow fixes him with a zero-degree-Kelvin glare. 'One in twenty women died in childbirth.'

Wednesday, 3 March 2010

Putting in the last of the skin staples after an uncompli-cated elective caesarean when the scrub nurse announces there's a discrepancy in the swab count – one's un-accounted for.* Don't panic, we tell ourselves, panicking. We check on the floor and inside the drapes – no swab. We rifle through the placenta and blood clots in the clinical waste bin like the world's most horrific bran tub – no swab. I call in Mr Fortescue, today's on-call con-sultant, to make the decision as to whether we re-open the patient or send her for an X-ray.†

Mr Fortescue decides we should re-open, and we wait for the anaesthetist's epidural top-up to take effect. He tells me a story from a few years ago: an elderly woman presented to him in clinic complaining of lower abdom-inal pain. After performing various other investigations, he sent her for an X-ray. The principal finding was the presence of a spoon in her abdominal cavity. After asking various pertinent questions – 'Have you ever eaten a spoon?', 'Do you stick spoons up your vagina or rectum?'

---

* For every operation, an inventoried set of instruments are used – and they are counted meticulously in and out. Swabs are packed together in stacks of five, and at the end of the procedure, the scrub nurse makes sure that she's discarding a total number of swabs that are a multiple of five so we know that none have been left inside the patient. (Unless five have somehow been left inside the patient.)

† Swabs are designed with a radio-opaque thread running through them as a marker, which show up on X-rays as a line. A bit un-imaginative – I'd have gone for a radio-opaque 'WHOOPS!'

– it seemed unlikely the origin of the object would be discovered. But it was causing her pain and needed to be removed at open surgery, under general anaesthetic.

Sure enough, at surgery, nestled among her intestines and other gizzards, was a dessert spoon. On removal, its only notable features were a number of scratches on the rear surface and the words 'Property of St Theodore's Hospital' stamped onto the handle. Mr Fortescue saw her on the ward post-operatively and they were each equally baffled as to how the spoon had somehow managed to backpack its way from St Theodore's into her abdominal cavity. Her last contact with them, save for their spoon stirring her innards like a risotto, was a caesarean section back in the 1960s. Some correspondence with St Theodore's followed, where they firmly denied the routine surgical implantation of spoons, but were able to dig out the patient's notes. They were unrevealing, spoon-wise – it seems very few doctors who empty canteens of cutlery into patients' stomachs are going to document it – but did provide the name of the surgeon. The gentleman was long since dead, but Mr Fortescue was eventually able to speak to someone who trained under him, to ask if his old boss was in the habit of breaking mid-caesarean for a spot of baked Alaska. Amazingly, this revealed the explanation. The surgeon in question routinely used a sterilized dessert spoon when sewing up the rectus sheath,* to protect underlying

---

* The rectus sheath is a fibrous layer underneath your abs – when

structures. On this occasion the spoon had clearly fallen in, and he'd just decided 'sod it' and ploughed on.

Our anaesthetist calls over that we're good to proceed, and as I start to remove the skin staples a midwife runs into theatre telling us to stop because the swab has been found: the baby was holding it. Much relief all round, except from the scrub nurse, who has been subjected to half an hour of unnecessary stress and bin-searching. 'The thieving little cunt,' she says – not seeing that directly behind the midwife is the swab in question, held by the baby in question, held by its father.

Thursday, 18 March 2010

A&E bleep urgently – a woman is delivering a baby at twenty-five weeks in a cubicle. Myself, SHO, anaesthetist and midwife peg it down to A&E, with the neonatal team following shortly behind, wheeling all their gubbins. She's huffing and puffing and in a terrible state – the anaesthetist gives her some pain relief. The midwife can't pick up a fetal heart with the Sonicaid – not good.

I examine the patient. She's not actively delivering. In fact her cervix is long, hard and closed – she's not in labour at all. This is odd. I ask where she's booked for this pregnancy and she says it's here. Someone looks

---

you sew it back up you need to be careful not to accidentally nick any of the underlying organs.

her up on the computer and there's nothing, not that this is unusual. The computer denies knowledge of almost every patient – we'd be better off with tarot cards.

One of the A&E staff scrambles to find me an ultrasound machine and I ask the patient when she had her most recent scan. Last week. This hospital, right? Yep. On the fifth floor? Yep. Ah, I see. I send the anaesthetist, midwife and paediatricians away. Any scans for patients here happen on the ground floor of this *three*-storey hospital.

The ultrasound machine appears, and luckily, given I've just sent away the rest of the team, there's no baby – just some distended loops of bowel making her look pregnant-ish. If you squint.

'But where's the baby? Where's it gone?' she screams to a packed and no doubt fascinated A&E department. I tell her my colleagues will be along shortly to explain, then ask A&E to contact psychiatry to kindly take over her management. I scoot over to the coffee shop for a sit-down and a quiet reflection on what I've just experienced. I'm cross other patients have been potentially endangered by her wolf-cry dragging so many clinicians away from labour ward. I'm baffled as to what she thought was going to happen – she knew she was about to get rumbled, right? And I'm sad for her – what kind of traumas and demons have taken her to a place where she does this? Hopefully my friends in psychiatry are currently giving her the help she needs.

Shame on me for thinking I'd be able to get through

a whole coffee undisturbed. I'm suddenly fast-bleeped to labour ward and run there as quickly as I can.

'Room four!' shouts the senior midwife as I wheeze onto the ward. It's the woman from A&E, huffing and puffing away again. She's clearly not giving up so easily and has absconded from A&E before her psychiatric review to try her luck elsewhere.

She sees me and looks extremely pissed off, parade well and truly rained upon.

Saturday, 27 March 2010

A nice evening out with a few old med school friends to persuade ourselves that our lives are fine, despite significant evidence to the contrary. It's nice to catch up, even if it needed to be rearranged seven times.

After dinner, we end up at the med school bar for old times' sake, and then for some reason, perhaps muscle memory from the last time we were there, start playing drinking games. The only game we can all remember the rules to is 'I have never'. It descends into therapy: all six of us have cried because of work, five of us have cried while at work, all of us have been in situations where we've felt unsafe, three of us have had relationships end because of work and all of us have missed major family events. On the plus side, three of us have had sex with nurses, and one of us while at work, so it's not all bad.

Monday, 19 April 2010

Miss Burbage, one of the consultants, has taken two weeks' compassionate leave because one of her dogs has died. Much piss-taking in the labour ward coffee room. I come to her defence, to everyone's surprise, not least my own.

Miss Burbage despises me – she decided I was hateful the moment she met me and hasn't budged from this standpoint. When I asked if I could get away from clinic early one evening for an anniversary dinner (earlier than it was going to end, not earlier than I was contracted to be there), she told me I should stay, on the grounds that I'd 'find it easier to get a new partner than a new job'. She told me if I expected to work in diabetic antenatal clinic, where I'd have to speak to patients about their diet, I'd need to have some self-respect and lose some weight (my BMI is 24). She has slapped my hand in theatre for holding a retractor incorrectly, and told me off for blasphemy after I said 'damn'. She has shouted in front of a patient that I'm an idiot and need to go back to med school.

And yet I'm sat defending her in front of my colleagues. Why make fun of someone for being upset? Surely this is cause to respect her – she knows everyone will find out her tough exterior was just that, an exterior. Shouldn't we feel sorry for someone who has so little else in their lives that they can be so totally floored by the death of their pet? Grief is grief – there's no right way and no normal. Mumblings of 'maybe' all round, and I wander off, having thoroughly suffocated that conversation with the pillow of my compassion. Two weeks for a dead dog though – the woman's fucking nuts.

Wednesday, 21 April 2010

One of the medical students saw me after a tutorial and asked me if I wouldn't mind taking a look at his penis. I did mind, but didn't really have much choice – it presumably takes quite a lot of nerve to ask one of your teachers to look at your dick. (Except in porn, where it seems to happen fairly regularly.) I took him into a side room and put on some gloves for the illusion of professionalism. He told me his penis was bruised and he'd had trouble urinating since last night.

It seemed there were certain elements of the story he'd omitted; his cock looked like an aubergine that had been attacked by a tiger – swollen, purple, and with deep oozing gashes down its entire length. On further questioning, I learned he was boasting to his girlfriend last night about the strength of his erections and announced to her that its throbbing robustness could stop the rotary blades of a desk fan. His hypothesis was monumentally incorrect and the desk fan proved the clear winner.

I suggested he attend A&E – a couple of the wounds needed closing and I suspected he might need catheterization until the swelling died down. And maybe go to a different hospital's A&E actually unless he fancied being known to his colleagues for the rest of his time here as Cock au Fan.[*]

Thursday, 22 April 2010

Perform my first cervical cerclage,[†] under the supervision of Prof. Carrow. In pretty much any other procedure, the consultant supervising you can slam his foot on the metaphorical dual controls at any point and stop you doing too much damage. But cerclage is all on you – they can talk you through it, but the tiniest slip with your stitch, anything but the steadiest hand, and you can rupture the membranes and end the pregnancy, doing exactly what the procedure is trying to prevent. And there's no way to practise the technique at home, like the way we learned to close wounds as house officers by cutting into an orange and sewing it back up.

Patient SW lost her first pregnancy at twenty weeks and is now thirteen weeks into her second. Prof. tells me to take it nice and slow, as steadily as I can. I'm aware

---

[*] Or Tony Fancock. Or Dick Fan Dyke. Or Knob-in-Fan Persie.

[†] Cervical cerclage is the treatment for cervical incompetence – a slightly horrible, cervix-shaming term for when the neck of the womb opens far too early in the pregnancy, causing late miscarriages or very pre-term births. The cerclage stitch is inserted during the first trimester of pregnancy and hopefully holds the cervix shut until just before full term.

that any shaking of my hand is magnified tenfold at the other end of the long needle-holding forceps, up by her cervix. Deep breaths, blink the sweat out of my eyes, one stitch, two, three, four, done. Got away with it.

I think it's the first time I've changed into a fresh pair of scrubs because my own sweat was the bodily fluid soaking me. It occurs to me scrubs are probably that shade of blue so patients can't see your sweat marks – a calm and professional demeanour is all well and good until the rapid darkening of your underarms betrays you.

Later, I realize there actually would be a way to practise the exact kind of small motor skills I need ahead of next time. I text my mum to ask if she by any chance still has that game of 'Operation' tucked away in a drawer.

She replies to say she's found it. She also has a Magic 8-Ball, she tells me, in case I need it for my diagnoses.

Saturday, 24 April 2010

Moral maze. Patient AB is in labour and has a non-reassuring trace. She's on her third midwife of the shift, having hurled racist abuse at the first two (black) midwives who had been looking after her. One more episode like that, she's been warned, and she'll be kicked off the labour ward. My SHO has reviewed the CTG and advises me that AB needs a caesarean section. Because I'm not entirely sure of the legality of following through with the threat to boot her out, the Indian SHO and I choose to ignore the fact that the patient has made racist comments to *her* too.

On reviewing the patient, I agree with the SHO – c-section it is. I transfer her to theatre and decide to stay tight-lipped about the fact I'm Jewish. The operation is straightforward, and a little boy is delivered safely (presumably to be immediately dressed up in 'Baby's First KKK Hood' and given a rattle in the shape of a burning cross).

But. If the patient had a dolphin tattoo on her right groin, would it be so bad if my skin incision was slightly wider than usual and I had no choice but to decapitate the dolphin? I could say, if pushed by an official inquiry (or some EDL henchman) that I'd been worried the baby was larger than average and it had made sense to have a good-sized operative field. And on closing the skin, would it be so bad if the wound didn't approximate very well for some strange, almost certainly unprovable reason, leaving the dolphin's head positioned a good inch to the left of its body?[*]

Saturday, 1 May 2010

I'm discussing a case with my colleague Padma in the coffee room after antenatal clinic, and a midwife leaps

---

[*] Well, we've spoken to a lawyer and the answer, it turns out, is, 'Yes. That would totally be assault.' So we'll say that I didn't do it.

into the conversation with, 'We actually don't like to use that word any more.' Wondering what outmoded terminology we've accidentally used (Consumption? Scrofula?), she lets us know that we said 'patient'. We should actually say 'client' – calling them patients is not only paternalistic and demeaning, but pregnancy is a normal and natural process rather than a pathological one. I just smile and remember the wise words taught to me by Mr Flitwick, one of my very first consultants, with regards to arguing with midwives – 'Do not negotiate with terrorists.'

Padma clearly has no such qualms. 'I had no idea *patient* was such a demeaning term,' she says. 'I'm so sorry, I'll never use it again. Client. Client's much better. Like what prostitutes have.'

Sunday, 9 May 2010

Having a poo on labour ward when the emergency buzzer goes off, and within minutes I've delivered a baby at crash caesarean section. The second the buzzer sounded I crimped it off, but my wiping was cursory at best, which is why my arse is now unbearably itchy while I'm scrubbed into theatre. It's acceptable to ask someone who's not scrubbed – a midwife or ODP – to push your mask or glasses up if they're falling off, or even to itch your nose. Would it be pushing it too far to ask them for a quick anal scratch?

Monday, 24 May 2010

I never volunteer my opinions on home births, but if, as today, a patient specifically asks me what I think of them, what I'd have if it were me, then I'll be honest. It's a five-minute speech, as follows: I tell them I don't doubt for a second that a home delivery that goes to plan must be a hundred times more calm, relaxing and pleasant than a hospital birth. (Though I'm not sure I could ever personally relax knowing that at any moment a blood and amniotic fluid emulsion might slosh onto the sofa. How would you go about getting that out?)

I then tell them I respect patient choice and that it's crucial they feel absolute ownership of their care. I tell them I get worried by the increasing promotion of 'natural' birth, and that demedicalization of pregnancy isn't necessarily a good thing – we should be proud of medical advances that objectively save lives, not scared of them.

I say I've seen a number of near misses, including one where we were seconds away from losing a child who'd been transferred to the labour ward when a home birth had gone pear-shaped. I also describe hospital deliveries I've seen in low-risk[*] mothers where rare and unpredictable events meant they or their baby would certainly have died outside of a hospital environment.

---

[*] On booking into antenatal clinic, patients are categorized as either high or low risk, and low-risk mothers are eligible for home births. People tend to forget that 'low risk' doesn't mean 'no risk'.

I promote midwife-based units, where women can have magical, wonderful births in more controlled environments. Crystals, beanbags, someone singing Radiohead songs backwards in Swedish – whatever floats your boat, just as long as you're a few hundred yards from a labour ward and their team of shit–fan separation specialists.

I acknowledge that when it comes to home births I only see the disasters and never the successes, which some people describe as a fatal flaw in my argument. Presumably they also have issues with firemen who advise the use of seatbelts, because they only see the drivers they angle-grind out of pile-ups, not the majority of safe car journeys. I will put my hand on my heart and tell the patient I implore anyone close to me to think twice about having a home delivery.

Unfortunately, today's clinic is running massively late, and I've got a dinner date, so I don't have time for all this. Instead, I give the abbreviated version: 'Home delivery is for pizzas.'

Wednesday, 2 June 2010

Teaching medical students this morning – they're keen to brush up on their X-ray reporting skills. I grab a couple of films from the trolley and shove one up on the light box. It's a normal chest X-ray of a patient, taken pre-operatively. The first student steps up to present.

'This is a PA chest radiograph taken yesterday of a

sixty-four-year-old female patient with name NW and date of birth 03/01/46. There is adequate inspiration and the film is well penetrated and not rotated.' He's good.

'The trachea is central, the mediastinum not displaced and the cardiac contours are normal. The obvious abnormality is a curvilinear mass in the superior lobe of the right lung, occupying . . .'

Hang on. Abnormality? Where the hell did that come from? Holy fuck. I reviewed this earlier and missed a tumour – I've sent the patient off to surgery and her certain death. I push past the student to get a better look at the cancer. Then I reposition the X-ray slightly and the mass moves. It was a 'Give Blood' sticker on the light box.*

Saturday, 5 June 2010

My life is starting to feel like an episode of *Quantum Leap*. I'll suddenly wake up and not know where I am

---

* My friend Percy was working as an orthopaedic SHO when there was a trauma call to A&E – a motorcyclist had flown off his bike and broken all sorts of bones. The chest X-ray (routinely performed to check lungs haven't been punctured), Percy was proud to announce, showed Varicella Pneumonia – a rare and dangerous complication of chicken pox with a characteristic X-ray appearance. The patient was clearly septic with this pneumonia, which caused him to lose control and fly off his bike. Or, as it eventually turned out, his lungs were fine – but loads of gravel had gone up the back of his jacket and shown up on the X-ray.

or what I have to do. Today, I startle awake to a loud knocking sound – I'm sitting in my car asleep at a set of lights and an old boy is rapping on the window with the handle of his umbrella, asking if I'm OK.

It's the second unexpected power nap of the night shift, after a scrub nurse tapped me on the shoulder while I was sat fast asleep on a theatre stool to tell me the patient was just being wheeled in for her marsupialization.* We're repeatedly reminded not to use empty patient side rooms to catch any sleep overnight – the management maintains we're paid to work full shifts. I want to ask the management if they've heard of that big ball of fire in the sky that makes it slightly harder to sleep during the day than at night? Or how easy they think it is to suddenly switch from working during the day and sleeping at night, to the exact opposite within twenty-four hours? But most of all I want to ask: if they or their wife needed an emergency caesarean section at 7 a.m., would they rather the registrar doing it had caught forty minutes' sleep when things were quiet, or had been forced to stay awake every second of the shift?

It's a surreal feeling being this tired – almost like being in a computer game. You're there but you're not there. I suspect my reaction times are currently the same

---

* Marsupialization is the treatment for a Bartholin's abscess – when the glands that provide vaginal lubrication become infected. You create a pouch to help the abscess drain – hence marsupialization, like a genital kangaroo.

as when I'm about three pints deep. And yet if I turned up at work pissed they'd probably be unimpressed – it's clearly important my senses are only dulled through exhaustion.

I left work at 9.30 a.m. – it took me an hour to write up the notes for my last caesarean because I was really struggling to find the words, like I was trying to bodge the sentences together in Spanish for my GCSE. Do the courts take this into consideration when you nod off and mow down an entire family on the way home?

Friday, 11 June 2010

I tell a woman in antenatal clinic that she has to give up smoking. She shoots me a look that makes me wonder if I've accidentally just said, 'I want to fuck your cat,' or, 'They're closing Lidl.' She refuses to entertain the idea of a smoking cessation class. I explain how bad smoking is for her baby, but she doesn't particularly seem to care – she tells me all her friends smoked through pregnancy and their kids are fine.

I'm tired and just want to go home. I look at the clock: it's half six, clinic was meant to end an hour ago and she's far from the last patient on my list. I snap.

'If you don't stop smoking when you're pregnant with a child then nothing on earth will stop you smoking, and you'll die of a smoking-related illness.' As I'm saying this I can hear it being repeated back to me slowly by a lawyer – I immediately apologize. But strangely, it seems to have worked – she looks at me like it's the first time she's ever truly listened to anyone, like she's about to stand on the chair and exclaim, 'O Captain! My Captain!' She doesn't, as luck would have it, because the chair doesn't look like it could take it, but she does ask me about those smoking cessation classes. Good to know that death threats are effective on my patients.

On her way out she jokes, 'Maybe I'll start heroin instead!' I laugh, and don't mention that yes, that would genuinely be safer for her unborn child.

Monday, 14 June 2010

Prof. Carrow is the consultant on call for labour ward today, which is about as much use as having a cardboard cutout of Cher on call for labour ward. In fact, Cardboard Cher might at least raise morale a bit.

You don't see Prof. Carrow during the day, you don't phone him at night – he's far too important for all that nonsense. When he appears on the ward this evening I can only assume that he's got lost or one of his first-degree relatives is currently giving birth.

It all falls into place as a documentary film crew show up behind him, cameras rolling.[*] 'Talk me through

---

[*] In London you're never more than six feet from a rat – and in a big hospital you're never more than six feet from a documentary film crew.

the labour ward board,' Carrow says to me, which I do. He nods along for the cameras. 'Sounds like you've got it all under control, Adam. But if you've got any problems at all during the night, just call me.' The crew have what they want and stop recording. Prof. doesn't miss a beat before saying, 'Obviously, don't.'

Tuesday, 15 June 2010

I've spent a lot of time with patient VF, as I've been performing FBSes* on her baby every hour. She and her husband have been having a blazing argument for the last four. It started with something about his parents, we've heard all about some friend's wedding where she was flirting with Chris *again* and now we're on to money. If I was at their dinner party I'd have secreted my uneaten pudding into a napkin, made my excuses and headed home ages ago, but I don't really have any choice but to eavesdrop. It's a thorough demonstration of the threadbare state of their relationship – I feel like

---

* Fetal Blood Sampling (FBS) is the most accurate way of checking baby's well-being – you lie mum on her side, stick a short length of guttering in her vagina and make a cut on the top of baby's head using a knife on a long stick. There's no pretending it's any more advanced than this. You then collect a drop of blood in a small capillary tube, and the midwife runs off to drop it, lose it, find that the machine is broken or occasionally report back with the pH of the baby's blood. For some reason they choose not to mention this fairly common procedure in antenatal classes.

a marriage counsellor who's been rendered completely mute.

In truth, they're behaving equally despicably, but given she's currently in labour – a famously non-fun process – I have to award him 100 per cent of the bastard points.

At one stage he goes out to take a phone call and the midwife quite rightly checks with VF that he's not been hitting her. She assures the midwife this isn't the case. He returns, the arguments continue, then escalate. He's puce-faced and yelling at her – we all ask him to either calm down or step out of the room. He screams at her, 'I never wanted this fucking baby anyway,' and storms out, never to reappear in the hospital. Jesus.

Friday, 18 June 2010

Patient RB presented to A&E with an ambulance crew and two police officers. And also, of note, a foot of metal pole protruding from her. She was being chased on foot by the police for some reason or other, and her escape plan involved climbing over some railings into a park. The escape plan unfortunately failed just as she was getting over the railings, when she slipped and one of the metal spikes slid up her vagina and penetrated through the front of her abdomen.

She'd had the presence of mind to get off her face on cocaine earlier in the evening, which anaesthetized her sufficiently until the Fire Brigade arrived on the scene and were able to cut off the railing just below vagina level (while presumably saying 'holy shit' quite a lot). She arrived here haemodynamically stable and remarkably well, all things considered, so we arranged an urgent CT to delineate precisely which cuts of meat were skewered on this particular kebab. Miraculously, she'd avoided damage to her bladder and major blood vessels, so it was just a case of taking her to theatre and sewing up the entry and exit wounds.

We reviewed her after surgery – sober, sore, embarrassed and with a police chaperone, as she was still under arrest. We told her that all looked well and gave her a post-operative management plan. She asked if she could keep the spike as a souvenir, and I said I couldn't see any reason why not. The policeman came up with a convincing one – it's really not a good idea to give an arrested criminal a weapon capable of piercing an abdomen.

Tuesday, 22 June 2010

What to do when you're managing an emergency and there's another emergency? I'm on labour ward when the buzzer goes off – mum's pushing and there's a horrendous-looking trace, baby needs to be urgently lifted out with forceps. I do the necessary and baby comes out quickly, but it's floppy. The paediatrician does her magic and the baby yelps to life. Placenta out and the patient is bleeding moderately, from a combination of the generous episiotomy[*] and a slightly boggy uterus. I start to do part two of the necessary when I hear another emergency buzzer. I'd better stay – this could quite easily escalate into a major PPH,[†] and in any case she's already losing blood every moment I'm not sewing her up or calling out the name of the next drug for the midwife to inject. On the other hand, this other unknown emergency could be much worse – and my current patient is very unlikely to suffer permanent harm if I leave her in the hands of an experienced midwife.

It's daytime, but who's to say all my colleagues aren't busy with patients, each assuming someone else will attend the emergency buzzer, which continues to sound. Or what if it's the kind of emergency that needs all hands on deck? I consider sending the midwife to report back, but that minute might be critical for the other patient. I hand the midwife a large swab and tell her to press hard on the perineal wound until I get back, and give her instructions about the next couple of drugs to get into the patient if necessary. I sprint out. The light is

---

[*] An episiotomy is a cut made with scissors (I'd love to say they were special surgical scissors but they're just normal scissors) into the perineum to prevent a tear that would be harder to repair or might go into the anus. Essentially, it's a controlled explosion.

[†] PPH means postpartum haemorrhage to half of all doctors and primary pulmonary hypertension to the other half, due to a naming ambiguity.

flashing outside room three and I bound in, hoping I've made the right decision. Naturally, I haven't.

A midwife is running a CPR drill. There's a mannequin on the bed and a bunch of doctors and nurses calling out what they'd do were this a real emergency. Which it isn't. Unlike the one I've just left. 'Right, the registrar is here,' says the midwife to the SHO. 'What would you like him to do?' What I in fact do is walk up to the mannequin, push it off the bed and call the midwife a cretin, accusing her of deliberately sabotaging patient safety. Then I bolt back to the first room, where all is thankfully stable, and get my non-imaginary patient as good as new. (OK, not quite.)

I clearly hadn't expressed my feelings adequately earlier, as the midwife supervisor takes me aside afterwards and asks me to apologize to the midwife in question for disrupting her simulation and upsetting her. My apology takes the shape of a clinical incident form, citing this simulation as a dangerous near miss. I'm sure I used to be nice before this job.

Wednesday, 23 June 2010

An email reminds us of the crucial importance of skills drills training for all clinical staff. However, before any drill is called, it is now policy to check all rooms to ensure no staff are otherwise engaged in emergencies.

Monday, 5 July 2010

A rare bit of continuity of care today. I saw this patient a month or so back in Miss Burbage's general gynae clinic, and it sounded very much like she had premature ovarian failure. Early menopause is rather beyond my scope, which I confessed to the patient, and excused myself while I left the room to speak to Miss Burbage for a management plan. She thought it was beyond her scope too, and it would be best to pop her into Mr Bryce's specialist endocrinology clinic in the next available slot. The patient wasn't too upset about the waste of her morning, knowing that she was getting to see the expert next time.

Today, however, I'm the registrar in Mr Bryce's endocrinology clinic, and he's off on holiday. Last time I saw the patient, I said I didn't have the faintest idea about her condition, and now she's sitting opposite me, having given up another afternoon to be here, expecting answers, needing help. Do I say I was just being modest last time? That I've been on a course since then? Do I put on an accent? Fake moustache?

I book her into clinic in a fortnight, when I know I'll be on nights, to avoid the possibility of a hat-trick.

Tuesday, 27 July 2010

Ron tried to dump me as a friend today – a proper, sombre, grown-up discussion. He doesn't know why he bothers trying to keep in touch with me when it's clear our lives have drifted apart massively since school.

I should at least vary up the excuses I give him. Do I really expect him to believe I couldn't come to his engagement party or his stag do because of work? That I couldn't make the wedding ceremony because of work, and almost missed the reception as well? That I missed his dad's funeral and his daughter's christening because of work? He knows my job's full-on, but how hard can it be to swap shifts if it's something you really want to do?

I put my hand on my heart and swear to Ron that I love him, he's one of my best friends and I wouldn't lie to him. I know I've been useless, but I've seen a lot more of him than almost anyone else I know – the job is just unimaginably busy. Non-medics can never appreciate quite how tough it is to be a doctor and the impact it has on real life. I totally lied about the christening, though – fuck that shit.

Monday, 2 August 2010

It's the final shift of the job – a night shift, naturally. My new post starts an hour before this one ends, about ten miles away – but I'll cross that bridge when I come to it, two hours late and bleary-eyed.

Technically this job ended at midnight, a fact that occurs to me on the stairwell at 12.10 a.m. when my swipe card refuses to let me back onto the ward and I realize it's been automatically deactivated. I'm Cinderella in scrubs.

If you ask the hospital to adequately staff a department, provide an effective computer system or even supply enough chairs for clinic, you'll get a shrug and a display of colossal incompetence. And yet when it comes to being able to get in and out of doors, they somehow take on the organizational skills of a cyborg librarian. If swipe cards suddenly start developing cancer, a cure will be found immediately.

I endure a mere quarter of an hour of banging on doors and praying the crash bleep doesn't go off before someone spots me and lets me back onto the ward.[*]

---

[*] The savvy obstetrician doesn't carry his mobile phone in his scrubs. All it takes is one iPhone to drown in a tsunami of blood for you to learn your lesson; and I can assure you that no amount of soaking it in rice will revive it.

9

Senior Registrar

Medicine is the host who manages to keep you at their party hours after you first think about leaving. 'Don't go before we've cut the birthday cake . . . You must meet Steve before you head off . . . I think Julie lives over your way – she's off home in a minute, why don't you go together . . .' Then before you know it you've missed the last train back and you're crashing on the sofa.

Having gone to medical school you might as well finish and become a house officer, then you might as well become an SHO, then you might as well become a registrar, then you might as well become a senior registrar and by then you're practically a consultant. There almost certainly don't need to be so many different grades; I strongly suspect it's designed so that the next step is always just round the corner. It's the £50 note you chase down the street, swept up by another gust of wind the millisecond before your hand makes contact. And it definitely works. One day I realized – as if blinking awake after a serious accident – that I was now in my thirties, still in a career I'd signed up for fourteen years earlier, based on the very flimsiest of reasons.

My ID card and salary now proudly said 'senior registrar' (although in fairness my salary also said 'bank cashier' or 'reasonably experienced milkman') and my next few postings would bridge the gap from junior doctor to consultant. And, in fact, life as a consultant looked pretty appealing. The pay goes up, the hours go down. Admin sessions, days off. No one forcing me to do urogynae clinics. My name in capital letters at the top of my parents' will (probably followed by 'he's a consultant gynaecologist, you know'). And, best of all, stability: a job that I can stay in as long as I want, where I don't have to pack my bags as soon as I've memorized the code on the changing-room door.

But first I had to get through my senior registrar posts – the storm before the calm. Yes, my registrar jobs had been manic and relentless, but this was a different kind of stress – now I was the highest-ranking person in the department out-of-hours. Knowing that when my bleep went off it was a problem that both the SHO and the registrar had failed to resolve. Knowing that if I couldn't deal with it, a mother or a baby might die. Having a consultant at home 'on call' is just a formality: most emergencies will be over in a matter of minutes, before they can even change out of their dressing gown. I would now need to accept ultimate responsibility for the fails and fuck-ups of an SHO and registrar I may have never met before. While I'd often go unbleeped for an hour or two on a night shift, I preferred to prowl anxiously around labour ward, flitting from room to room asking 'Is everything OK?', suffering the occasional flashback to that registrar who told me as a student that obs and gynae was an easy speciality. Lying bastard.

So it wasn't the biggest surprise in the world when I registered with a GP and the practice nurse recorded my blood pressure as 182/108 mmHg.* She wouldn't accept my explanation that I was just off a night shift with two locums, still tightly wound from twelve hours on the wards, my mind jittering with a dozen medical equivalents of 'Did I turn the gas off?' Did the patient have that CT scan? Did I put in a second layer of stitches? Did I prescribe that methotrexate?

She booked me back in to see the GP the following week, and it was just as high. Again, I was straight back from work. I assured her I'd checked it myself in clinic and it was completely normal, but she wanted to be sure, just the same. In fairness to her, I was totally lying: I'd done no such thing. She arranged for me to have twenty-four-hour ambulatory monitoring.† Because days

---

* You'd want your blood pressure to be under 120/80 mmHg, aka millimetres of mercury. If you stuck a glass tube full of mercury into your heart, it's the number of millimetres the pressure would push the level up – though these days we use a slightly less invasive method to measure it. The top number is the pressure when your heart is going 'lub', the bottom number is when it's going 'dub'.

† Ambulatory monitoring involves wandering round with a blood-pressure cuff on your arm for a day, which inflates every fifteen mins or so and records the data for the doctor. It's particularly useful in 'white coat hypertension' when patients get nervous on visiting the doctor, so their BP rockets up whenever it's measured. About a week before finals at medical school, my friend Antonin asked during a

off work were in short supply, I wore it on an antenatal clinic day, making it practicable (I won't have to go to theatre) plus theoretically low stress. I sat in clinic and explained to patients that I needed to start them on antihypertensive medication, despite the device strapped to my arm proudly displaying that my blood pressure was significantly higher than theirs.

Among all the predictably 'hilarious' remarks the patients made to me, one said something surprisingly astute. 'It's funny – you don't think of doctors getting ill.' It's true, and I think it's part of something bigger: patients don't actually think of doctors as being human. It's why they're so quick to complain if we make a mistake or if we get cross. It's why they'll bite our heads off when we finally call them into our over-running clinic room at 7 p.m., not thinking that we also have homes we'd rather be at. But it's the flip side of not wanting your doctor to be fallible, capable of getting your diagnosis wrong. They don't want to think of medicine as a subject that anyone on the planet can learn, a career choice their mouth-breathing cousin could have made.

After an hour at home, my blood pressure returned to normal, so mercifully my arteries were still in decent nick. Plus it was interesting to be able to quantify in millimetres of mercury precisely how stressful it was to be a senior registrar.

---

tutorial, 'Why's it called *white goat hypertension*?' He's a consultant haematologist now if you want to watch out for him.

Monday, 9 August 2010

A patient named their baby after me today. It was a planned caesarean for breech presentation, and after I delivered the baby I said, 'Adam's a good name.' The parents agreed, and job's a good 'un.

I say 'Adam's a good name' after every single baby I deliver, and this was the first time that anyone's ever said yes. I've not even had a middle name before. But today this wrong was righted, and the squad of Adams I so richly deserve was launched in theatre two. (I'm not sure what I'll do with this team once they're assembled. Fight crime, maybe? Get them to cover my shifts?)

The SHO assisting me in the caesarean asked how many babies I've delivered. I estimated 1,200. He then looked up some population data and told me that on average 9 of every 1,200 babies born in the UK would be called Adam. I have genuinely put off eight sets of parents from naming their child after me.

Sunday, 15 August 2010

Summoned to a delivery room by one of the junior registrars – she's struggling to lock a pair of forceps onto the baby's head. We've had the occasional set of mismatched pairs sent to us recently – two left sides or

slightly different models packed together after sterilization. On examination, the left blade is placed well on the
side of baby's head. The right blade, however, is wedged
halfway up the patient's rectum.

Mistake corrected and baby delivered safely. (By me
– at this point I wouldn't trust the registrar to deliver a
limerick.)

'Do we have to tell her?' she asks conspiratorially,
testing my ethical boundaries like I'm a builder and she's
hoping to avoid the VAT.

'Of course not,' I say. '*You* do.'

Monday, 23 August 2010

Week three of the job and I'm just about up to speed
with the infertility* treatment eligibility criteria here.
Today I saw a couple who've had an unsuccessful round
of IVF – which was unsurprising. Chances of success in
their particular case were around 20 per cent for a single
cycle. Where I worked a month ago, a walkable distance
away, they'd have qualified for three cycles, which
would have upped their odds to nearer 50 per cent. They
ask me what private treatment would cost and I tell
them – around four thousand pounds for a cycle. The

---

* Infertility clinic got rebranded to 'subfertility clinic' during the
course of my training to make it sound less negative, and then again
to 'fertility clinic', which feels a bit 'la la la this isn't happening'
fingers-in-ears-y. Unless over in oncology they're now running the
'definitely not got breast cancer' clinic?

look on their faces tells me I may as well have said four trillion pounds.*

People say it's a choice to have kids, which is of course true. But no one argues that patients with recurrent miscarriages shouldn't be allowed treatment until they have a baby – and the NHS rightly doesn't limit their care. And how about the patient who had two ectopic pregnancies, leaving her with no fallopian tubes and no chance of getting pregnant without IVF? All we're doing is allowing people to make a choice they would have otherwise had were it not for a medical condition. Or not, because their surname begins with the letter G. I'm exaggerating of course – that would be ridiculous. They'd only be denied it for sensible reasons, such as living one road outside of an arbitrary catchment area.

I suggest they take a bit of a break to think about their options and come to terms with their feelings. I

---

* In most aspects of private medicine, you get a mild upgrade on the NHS, but no huge difference in actual care. You get seen a bit quicker, the receptionist's got all her teeth and there's a decent wine list for your inpatient stay – but ultimately you get the same treatment. When it comes to infertility medicine though, the private sector is leagues ahead – they will investigate and treat you until you have a baby (or an insolvency order). The NHS requires you to fit into quite a narrow demographic to qualify for any treatment, and it's often not enough to achieve a positive result. I understand there's a limited pot of money, but you don't ever hear this said in other corners of medicine. 'We don't treat leukaemia – there's a limited pot of money.' 'We only treat fractures on the right side of the body – there's a limited pot of money.'

float the possibilities of fostering or adoption. 'It's not the same though, is it?' the husband says, and no, it's probably not.

In the short time I've been working here I've told a lesbian couple they are eligible for treatment but a gay male couple wanting surrogacy that they're not. I've told a woman she's too old for treatment according to our criteria, even though she wasn't too old when she was referred here a few months ago. (And wouldn't have been too old a few streets away.) I've been cast in the role of a malevolent god.

Here there's a BMI limit for receiving treatment – something I've never encountered before. I had to tell a patient she was three kilos too heavy to be referred for IVF and to see me again when she'd lost the weight. She burst into tears, so I accidentally recorded her weight on the form as a few kilos too light.* Last week I wrote a letter citing exceptional circumstances, requesting treatment be allowed for a woman who had a child from a previous relationship who died in infancy, which cruelly makes her ineligible for treatment here.

I leave clinic, passing a rack of leaflets that details all the different fertility treatment options that the NHS in this area makes it all but impossible to receive. We should be more honest and replace them all with one called, 'Have you thought about getting a cat?'

---

* Is this the 'one weird weight-loss trick that doctors don't want you to know about' much vaunted by internet adverts?

Wednesday, 25 August 2010

An eighty-five-year-old, long-stay gynae oncology patient broke our hearts on yesterday's ward round. She misses her late husband, her children have barely visited since she's been in hospital and she can't even have her usual whiskey nightcap in here. I decided to play Boy Scout, prescribed whiskey (50 ml nightly) on her drug chart and gave the house officer £20 to get a bottle from the supermarket to pass on to the nursing staff, so they can fulfil the prescription on their drug round.

This morning, the ward sister reports that the patient declined her drink because, and I quote: 'Jack Daniel's is fucking cat piss.'

Monday, 13 September 2010

A new midwife supervisor, Tracy, has started this week and seems absolutely lovely – calm, experienced and sensible. She is now the second midwife supervisor on the unit called Tracy, the current one being a flappy, angry nightmare. To avoid confusion, we have nicknamed them 'Reassuring Trace' and 'Non-reassuring Trace'.

Friday, 24 September 2010

Moral maze. A *Crackerjack* bleep from theatre – it's Friday, it's five to five, it's something enormously time-consuming. Today's contestant is an emergency ectopic, and theatre would like me to pop up now. This is particularly annoying timing as it's date night. In fact, it's more than date night. It's date night somewhere extremely expensive to apologize for half-a-dozen recently cancelled date nights and to paper over the widening fault lines in our relationship. It's D-Date night. I should be fine if I leave by 6 p.m., I tell myself. At 5.45 it's time to start operating. The evening registrar is stuck in A&E and can't relieve me.

Best practice is to operate laparoscopically – about an hour's work for me, it leaves the patient with a couple of tiny holes and she'll be home tomorrow. Alternatively, I can make a quick incision in this twenty-five-year-old's pristine abdomen and sentence her to a proper scar and a longer hospital stay – but get away on time and keep my relationship on track. Besides, maybe the patient likes hospital food? I hesitate for a moment more, then request the laparoscopy set.

Tuesday, 5 October 2010

On the phone to my friend Sophia, having a moan about the levels of exhaustion and demoralization in our hospitals. We're both pretty fed up. She tells me she's just got her private pilot's licence and is planning to take a break from the NHS. 'And work for an airline?' I ask.

Actually, she's going to charter an aircraft and fly it around twenty-four African countries, visiting remote areas where maternal morbidity is the highest and teaching the local midwives some life-saving techniques. She'll also donate huge amounts of medical supplies and educational resources which she's going to fundraise for before she sets off. Now I feel exhausted, demoralized and selfish.

Monday, 11 October 2010

A text out of the blue from Simon; no news has been good news for the last eighteen months so my heart rather sinks when I see his name pop up. He's just asking for my address – he wants to send me a wedding invitation. I'm choked up that he'd think of me, and very much looking forward to intending to go, then pulling out at the last minute due to work.

Tuesday, 12 October 2010

The final patient of a comically busy antenatal clinic requests an elective caesarean section because of a previous traumatic vaginal delivery. This is a fairly common request – principally because there's no such thing as a non-traumatic vaginal delivery. The SHO who saw her last did the sensible thing and requested the notes from the hospital where she had her last baby, and I skim through them to see if anything particularly traumatizing had happened.

She had a long labour, resulting in a forceps extraction, and needed repair in theatre afterwards for a cervical tear. That night, she had a gargantuan post-partum haemorrhage, which caused her to arrest. She was successfully resuscitated – clearly, given she's sitting in clinic – and was taken back to theatre to resew her tear. This second attempt – almost unbelievably – went even worse and resulted in damage to her small bowel, and ultimately to a small bowel resection and stoma formation. Then a series of clinic letters from psychiatry, documenting her gradual recovery from PTSD caused by these events, and the collapse of her marriage. And now she's back to do it again. The woman must be so hard you can skate on her; let her have what she wants.

I book her in for an elective section. It's nice to have the bar set so low that almost anything we do will be a considerable upgrade on last time.

Thursday, 14 October 2010

I was slightly weirded out the first time a patient started texting during an internal examination, but now it seems reasonably common. Today, during a smear test, a patient FaceTimed her friend.

Sunday, 17 October 2010

I attend an emergency buzzer late at night – it's a shoulder dystocia.[*]

---

[*] Shoulder dystocia is one of the scariest experiences as an obstetri-

It's clearly a big baby, quadruple-chinned through how tightly its neck is being squeezed back against mum's perineum – and it's an experienced midwife, who I know will have already tried everything in the book. There's no pretending to the patient this isn't serious, but she's a dream so far – remaining calm and going along with everything asked of her.

I drain the bladder with a catheter, put her legs in McRoberts' position, apply suprapubic pressure. This is like no shoulder dystocia I've dealt with before. There's no give at all; the baby isn't budging. I ask the midwife supervisor to see if there are somehow any obstetric consultants in the building. I attempt Wood's Screw manoeuvre: nothing. I attempt to deliver the posterior arm: impossible. I roll the patient onto all fours and try all the manoeuvres again in this position. I ask the midwife to get my consultant on the phone. It's approaching five minutes of shoulder dystocia and something needs to happen urgently if the baby's going to live.

As I see it, I have three options as last-ditch attempts. The first is Zavanelli's manoeuvre – push the baby's

---

cian – the baby's head delivers, but the shoulders get stuck. All the time this is going on, baby's brain isn't getting any oxygen, so it's a ticking time bomb of a matter of minutes before irreversible brain damage occurs. We all train regularly in how to manage this particular emergency. Embedded into our brainstems are all manner of mnemonics to help us through it, and all sorts of physical manoeuvres: exerting suprapubic pressure, McRoberts (hyper-flexing the legs), Wood's Screw (rotating the baby by its shoulders), delivering the posterior arm.

head back inside and perform a crash caesarean section. I've never seen it done but I'm confident I can manage it. I'm also fairly confident that by the time we get her delivered in theatre the baby will have died.

Second option is to intentionally fracture baby's clavicle to allow baby to deliver. I have never seen this done either, and have no real idea how to go about it – it's a famously difficult procedure, even in much better hands than mine.

Third option is to perform a symphisiotomy, cutting the mother's pubic bone to make the outlet bigger. Again, I've never seen it performed, but I'm sure I can do it easily, and that it will be the quickest way to get the baby out. I inform the consultant over the phone that this is what I'm going to do – she checks what I've tried so far and confirms my understanding of how to perform it. She's driving in from home, but we both know that by the time she arrives everything will be over, one way or the other.

I feel as sick as I've ever felt in a clinical situation: I'm about to break a patient's pelvis and it might already be too late for her baby. Before I take the scalpel to her I have one last attempt to deliver the baby's posterior arm. All the various manoeuvres and shifts in position have somehow made something budge, and the arm delivers, followed by a very limp baby, who the midwife passes to the paediatricians. As we wait for the cry that may or may not come, I remember an old phrase in the textbooks that describes a successful shoulder dystocia delivery as 'greater strength of muscle or some infernal juggle' and totally get what the author was on about. The baby cries. Hallelujah. The midwife bursts into tears. We will have to wait and see if there's an Erb's,[*] but the paediatrician whispers in my ear that both arms seem to be behaving normally.

I see that I've given the mother a third-degree tear, which isn't ideal, but is pretty minor collateral damage in the grand scheme of things. I ask the midwife to prepare her for theatre – that'll give me twenty minutes to write up my delivery notes and grab a cup of coffee. My SHO comes in – can I quickly do a ventouse extraction in another room?

Wednesday, 20 October 2010

Maybe it's because his first language is Greek. Maybe he's forgotten our previous discussion where I'd offered to help him with ultrasound technique. Maybe I should have phrased it as 'determine fetal gender'. But judging by the SHO's look of confusion and disgust and his hasty retreat down the corridor, what I shouldn't have said was a cheery, 'Would you like to watch me sex a baby?'

---

[*] Erb's palsy is nerve damage to the arm resulting from straining the neck in this kind of scenario.

Thursday, 21 October 2010

I pick up notes for the next patient I'm seeing in gynae clinic. I recognize the name – flicking through the notes, I see a clinic letter I wrote to her GP back in March. I spot a horrifying typo in my sign-off, thanks to a missing 'hesitate to'.

> *If you have any questions whatsoever, please do not contact me.*

It worked, though. Not a peep.

Wednesday, 27 October 2010

I'm in occupational health for a follow-up HIV test after a needle-stick injury from a positive patient three months ago. She had an undetectable viral load but it's still not ideal by any stretch, and I've had it constantly in the back of my mind since, like a bill from HMRC.

Making nervous small talk with the occupational health registrar as he takes my blood, I ask what happens to an obstetrician who's HIV positive. 'You wouldn't be able to do clinical procedures, so no labour ward, theatre, on-calls – just clinics, I guess.' I don't say it, but that would really take the sting out of the diagnosis.[*]

---

[*] Since 2013, it's been OK for an HIV-positive doctor with an undetectable viral load to operate, after a decade of lobbying that the

Sunday, 31 October 2010

At a friend's Halloween party I spot someone I know from somewhere. School, I think.

I amble over to say hi. Blank face. Not school. University? Nope.

Where did you grow up? Have we worked together? Humiliatingly for me, but probably for his own sanity, he has to stop me and say that I've probably just seen him on TV before – he's a presenter called Danny. Humiliatingly for *him*, I say the name maybe rings a bell, but I'm pretty sure that's not it. His wife wanders over and I work it out – I delivered their baby by caesarean a year or so back.

Much hugging, hand-shaking and what-a-coincidence-ing. Danny jokes he's glad it was a caesarean, because he doesn't know how he'd feel about talking to a man who's seen his wife's vagina. I want to say that *actually* I'd have seen it when catheterizing her for the procedure, plus, if he really wants something to get his brain imploding, I'd have also seen its reverse side during the operation. I don't say this, just in case he wasn't joking and things get even more awkward.

---

risk to patients was negligible. My blood test was negative, in case you wondered whether the book was about to take a dark turn.

Monday, 8 November 2010

The cherry on top of a record-breakingly hellish night shift (with a locum registrar who was of barely more than ornamental value) was a crash caesarean at 7.45 a.m., fifteen minutes from the supposed finish line. Caesarean, then another caesarean, then ventouse, then forceps, then caesarean, then I lost count, but a bunch more babies, and now a final caesarean. I'm absolutely exhausted, and would gladly have dragged my feet and handed it over to the morning shift were the trace not pre-terminal.*

I've not sat down for twelve hours, let alone rested my eyes, my dinner's sitting uneaten in my locker and I've just called a midwife 'Mum' by accident. We run to theatre and I deliver the baby very quickly – it's limp, but the paediatricians do their black magic and soon it's making the right sort of noises. Cord gases confirm we made the right decision and I close up the patient on a vague high.

The paediatrician grabs me for a word after I leave theatre and tells me I've cut the baby's cheek with my scalpel while making the uterine incision – it's not bad, but just to let me know. I go straight to see the baby and parents. It's not a deep cut, nor is it long – it didn't need any skin closure and it surely won't scar – but it was totally my fault. I apologize to the parents, who couldn't

---

* Pre-terminal means the baby is about to die if nothing is done.

248

seem to give less of a toss. They're in love with their gorgeous (and only mildly mutilated) little girl, and they tell me they understand she had to be delivered in a bit of a rush – these things happen. I want to say that these things aren't meant to happen, that they haven't happened to me before and they almost certainly wouldn't have happened to me at the start of the shift.

I offer them a leaflet with the details of the PALS office – they don't want it. A close shave for my GMC registration and an actual shave for the poor baby. A couple of centimetres higher and I'd have taken her eye out, a couple of millimetres deeper and I could have caused scarring and blood loss. Babies have even died from lacerations at caesarean. I document our discussion in the notes, fill in the clinical incident form, do everything demanded of me by the system that allowed this to happen in the first place. Before long I'll get sat down by someone to be gently or not-so-gently chastised, and at no point will it occur to them that there might be a more fundamental problem here.*

Thursday, 11 November 2010

I suspected the husband of the couple in infertility clinic had a urinary tract infection so I gave him a specimen

---

* Almost a decade previously, I worked at the same hospital as a medical secretary during university holidays. We were obliged to take a twenty-minute break after every two hours of staring at a computer screen because of 'health and safety'.

pot and sent him off to the toilet for a sample. He took the jar from me and peered at it for a few seconds before tottering off. I suppose it was my fault for not being specific enough, but he returned (admirably quickly) with the pot containing a few millilitres of semen. The miscommunication could have been worse, of course – he could've shat in it, bled into it or stuck a skewer into the ventricles of his brain to draw out a pot of cerebro-spinal fluid. I do rather wonder whether the reason they're struggling to conceive is that he's urinating into his wife during sex.

Sunday, 14 November 2010

It's Sunday lunchtime and patient RZ needs a caesarean section for failure to progress in labour. The patient is happy to have a section, but her husband doesn't want me to perform it because I'm male. They are orthodox Muslim and have apparently been told they can have all female doctors. I say I don't know who told them that but, although there are often women doctors available, we work on a rota and currently the entire team in obs and gynae is male, including the consultant on call at home.

'So you're honestly telling me that there are no female doctors in the hospital?'

'No, sir, I'm telling you there are no female doctors in the hospital capable of performing a caesarean. I'm sure I could easily find your wife a female dermatologist.'

The patient is clearly much happier with the idea of me doing the section than her husband is, but she's not really being allowed to speak up. We go through the motions, getting even further away from the result we need the more we dance around it. 'When's a woman doctor next here?' When the shifts change in seven hours, which would be a very bad idea for your baby. 'Can't the midwife do it?' No, and nor can the cleaner.

I call the consultant for some moral support. He suggests I drag up, and I suspect he's only half joking. Back in the room, I ask, 'Does the Koran not allow for male doctors to operate in the case of an emergency?' Which, I remind them, this is. It's a total bluff, but it seems the sort of thing a religious text might say. They ask me to give them five minutes, make some phone calls, then the husband comes to find me to say that they're happy for me to deliver the baby. He says it in a way that implies I should be grateful. In fact, I am grateful, but only because my main concern was the safe appearance of his child, not his (or anyone else's) God's feelings on the matter. Plus I don't have a Plan B and can't begin to contemplate the unending quantity of paperwork that would otherwise haunt me forever.

The (male, naturally) anaesthetist pops in to get them sorted for theatre, and I wonder whether this will be a growing trend. Perhaps we should take a leaf from toilet cleaners and litter the floor with yellow 'Male Obstetrician on Duty' signs.

Before long we're in theatre, and I've safely delivered

their baby girl. Healthy mum, healthy baby – it's all we ever aim for, and they should be glad everything worked out fine for them, when it doesn't for so many families who come through these doors.

In the event, the husband is extremely thankful – he apologizes for wasting my time and adding to my stress, and tells me he's grateful for all I've done. As with most husbands who kick off, he was probably just stressed by the situation, and I presume the added jeopardy of potential eternal damnation didn't help either.

He's going down to the shops, would I like anything? I half want to see his reaction if I ask for a BLT, a bottle of Smirnoff and some poppers.

Thursday, 18 November 2010

Was meant to be back home at 7 p.m. sharp but it's 9.30 and I've only just come off labour ward. Feels appropriate that work commitments mean I have to reschedule collecting all my belongings from the flat. On the plus side, my depressing new bachelor pad is only ten minutes from the hospital.

Monday, 22 November 2010

A patient awaiting review in A&E for some minor abdominal pain has sunk lower and lower down my list of priorities throughout the afternoon as labour ward has become busier and busier. I'm in the middle of stabilizing a patient with severe pre-eclampsia when I'm bleeped by a furious A&E registrar.

'If you don't come to A&E right now this patient is going to breach the four-hour target.'*

'OK. But if I *do* come right now my current patient is going to die.' Mic drop.

There's a good five seconds of radio silence where he clearly wonders if there's anything he can fire back that will persuade me to come down and save him a load of aggro. I spend this time marvelling at a system that's so obsessed with arbitrary targets that his reply should take this long to generate.

'Fine. Just come when you can,' he replies. 'But I'm really not happy about this.' When she's out of the woods I must remember to have my pre-eclamptic patient write him an apology.

Friday, 26 November 2010

The last of my pre-operative patients to consent before theatre is QS, an elderly lady having a hysteroscopy following some recent PV bleeding. She's accompanied by

---

* Because hospitals aren't under quite enough pressure, the government has decided that all patients in A&E need to be admitted or discharged within four hours, whether they've had a stroke or stubbed their toe. If more than 5 per cent of these patients breach the target (unfortunately not the type of breech that interests me), the hospital gets fined and the management unleash a heap of hell on the A&E staff.

a red-trousered roaring chin of a son. He's under the impression that the more he treats medical staff like crap, the more convinced they will be of his importance, and thus the better treatment they will receive. Amazingly, this is a commonly held belief and, annoyingly, he's absolutely right. People like this are exactly the type to complain to PALS if she gets so much as a chip in her toenail polish.

I bite my tongue harder with every question he asks. 'How many of these have you done?' 'Is this not a case that your consultant should be doing?' If this was a restaurant and I was a waiter, I would currently be stirring my spit and semen into his beef bourguignon; but she's a sweet old lady, and she's not going to suffer just because her son's an arsehole. We're all done. 'Treat her as if she's your own mother,' he instructs me. I assure him he really doesn't want *that* at all.

Sunday, 5 December 2010

Spending my Sunday afternoon on labour ward with an excellent SHO. She asks me to review the CTG of a patient and I agree with her assessment that the patient needs a caesarean section for fetal distress. They are a lovely couple, recently married; it's their first baby, and they understand the situation.

The SHO asks if she can perform the caesarean while I assist. In theatre, the SHO goes through the layers: skin, fat, muscles, peritoneum 1, peritoneum 2, uterus. After the uterine incision, rather than amniotic fluid, blood comes out – lots of blood. There has been an abruption.[*] I stay calm and ask the SHO to deliver the baby – she says she can't, there's something in the way. I take over the operation – the placenta is in the way. The patient has an undiagnosed placenta praevia. This should have been noticed on scans, she should never have been allowed to go into labour. I deliver the placenta and then deliver the baby. The baby is clearly dead. Paediatricians attempt resuscitation but without success.

The patient is bleeding heavily from the uterus – one litre, two litres. My sutures have no effect, drugs have no effect. I call for the consultant to come in urgently. The patient is now under general anaesthetic and receiving emergency blood transfusions; her husband has been escorted out of theatre. Blood loss is now five litres. I try a brace suture[†] – no luck. I'm squeezing the uterus as hard as I can with both hands – it's the only thing that stops the bleeding.

The consultant arrives, attempts another brace suture – it doesn't work. I see the panic in her eyes. The anaesthetist tells us he can't get fluid into the patient fast enough to replace what she's losing and we're risking

---

[*] Abruption is a complication of pregnancy where all or part of the placenta separates from the uterus. Because all of baby's oxygen and nutrients are delivered via the placenta, this can be extremely serious indeed.

[†] Brace sutures are very large stitches that go around the uterus like a pair of braces to compress it and stop the bleeding.

organ damage. The consultant calls another colleague –
he's not on duty, but he's the most experienced surgeon
she can think of. We take it in turns squeezing the uterus
until he arrives twenty minutes later. He performs a hysterectomy; the bleeding is finally under control. Twelve
litres. The patient goes to intensive care and I am warned
to expect the worst. My consultant talks to the husband.
I start to write up my operation notes but instead just
cry for an hour.

10

Aftermath

That was the last diary entry I wrote, and the reason there aren't any more laughs in this book.

Everyone at the hospital was very kind to me and said all the right things; they told me it wasn't my fault, said I couldn't have done anything differently, and sent me home for the rest of the shift. And yet, at the same time, it felt a bit like I'd sprained my ankle. A flurry of people asking me, 'Are you OK?', but also the definite expectation that I'd still come into work the next day, the reset button firmly pressed. That's not to say they were heartless or unthinking – it's a problem that's baked into the profession. You can't wear a black armband every time something goes wrong, you can't take a month's compassionate leave – it happens too often.

It's a system that barely has enough slack to allow for sick leave, let alone something as intangible as recovering from an awful day. And, in truth, doctors *can't* acknowledge how devastating these moments really are. If you're going to survive working in this profession, you have to convince yourself these horrors are just part of your job. You can't pay any attention to the man behind the curtain – your own sanity relies on it.

I'd seen babies die before. I'd dealt with mothers on the brink of death before. But this was different. It was the first time I was the most senior person on the ward when something terrible happened, when I was the person everyone was relying on to sort it all out. It was on me, and I had failed.

Officially, I hadn't been negligent and nobody suggested otherwise. The GMC will always judge medical negligence by asking the question, 'Would your peers have done anything differently in that situation?' All my peers would have done exactly the same things and had exactly the same outcome. But this wasn't good enough for me. I knew that if I'd been better – super-diligent, super-observant, super-something – I might have gone into that room an hour earlier. I might have noticed some subtle changes on the CTG. I might have saved the baby's life, saved the mother from permanent compromise. That 'might have' was inescapable.

Yes, I came back to work the next day. I was in the same skin, but I was a different doctor – I couldn't risk anything bad ever happening again. If a baby's heart rate dropped by one beat per minute, I would perform a caesarean. And it would be me doing it, no SHOs or junior registrars. I knew women were having unnecessary caesareans and I knew colleagues were missing opportunities to improve their surgical skills, but if it meant everyone got out of there alive it was worth it. I'd mocked consultants for being over-cautious before, rolled my eyes the moment they turned their heads, but now I got it. They'd each had their own 'might have' moment, and this is how you dealt with it.

Except, I wasn't *really* dealing with it, I was just getting on with it. I went six months without laughing, every smile was just an impression of one – I felt bereaved. I should have had counselling – in fact, my hospital should have arranged it. But there's a mutual code of silence that keeps help from those who need it most.

No matter how vigilant I was, another tragedy would have happened eventually. It has to – you can't prevent the unpreventable. One brilliant consultant tells her trainees that by the time they retire there'll be a bus full of dead kids and kids with cerebral palsy, and that bus is going to have their name on the side. A huge number of 'adverse outcomes', as they say in hospital-ese, will occur on their watch. She tells them if they can't deal with that, they're in the wrong profession. Maybe if someone had said that to me a bit earlier I'd have thought twice. Ideally, back when I was choosing my A levels and getting myself into this mess.

I asked if I could go part-time ('not unless you're pregnant') and investigated switching to general practice. But first I'd have to drop right down to SHO grade for a couple of years to work in A&E, paediatrics and psychiatry. I didn't want to take a long journey backwards in order to start moving forwards again, only to find I didn't like that either.

I paused my training with the deanery and did some half-hearted research and lazy locum shifts on private units, but after a few months I hung up my stethoscope. I was done.

I didn't tell anyone the reason why I left. Maybe I should have; maybe they'd have understood. My parents reacted like I'd told them I was being tried for arson. At first I *couldn't* talk about it, then it became something I just *didn't* talk about. When cornered, I would reach for my red nose and clown horn, and bring out my anecdotes about objects in anuses and patients 'saying the funniest things'. Some of my closest friends will read this book and hear that story for the first time.

These days, the only doctoring I do is other people's words – I write and script-edit comedy for television. A bad day at work now is if my laptop crashes or a terrible sitcom gets terrible ratings – stuff that literally doesn't matter in the scheme of things. I don't miss the doctor's version of a bad day, but I do miss the good days. I miss my colleagues and I miss helping people. I miss that feeling on the drive home that you've done something worthwhile. And I feel guilty the country spent so much money training me up for me just to walk away.

I still have a very strong affinity with the profession – you never totally stop being a doctor. You still run to the injured cyclist sprawled across the road, you still reply to the text messages from friends of friends cadging fertility advice. So in 2016, when the government started waging war on doctors – forcing them to work harder than ever for less money than ever – I felt huge solidarity with them. And when the government repeatedly lied that doctors were simply being greedy, that they do medicine for the money – for anything other than the best interests of the patient – I was livid. Because I knew it wasn't true.

The junior doctors lost that particular battle, largely because the government's booming, baleful voice drowned out their own reasonable, experienced, quiet one. I realized that every healthcare professional – every single doctor, nurse, midwife, pharmacist, physio and paramedic – needs to shout about the reality of their work, so the next time the health secretary lies that doctors are in it for the money, the public will know just how ridiculous that is. Why would any sane person do that job for anything other than the right reasons? Because I wouldn't wish it on anyone. I have so much respect for those who work on the front line of the NHS because, when it came down to it, I certainly couldn't.

Putting this book together, six years after quitting medicine, I met up with dozens of former colleagues. Their dispatches from labour ward tell of an NHS on its knees. Every one of them spoke of an exodus from medicine. When I left, I was a glitch in the matrix, an aberration. Now every rota bears the scars of doctors who've activated their Plan B – working in Canada or Australia, in pharmaceutical companies or in the City. Most of my old colleagues were themselves desperately groping for a ripcord to parachute out of the profession – brilliant, passionate doctors who've had their reasons to stay bullied out of them by politicians. Once upon a time, these people were rescheduling their own weddings for this job.

The other recurrent theme, doctor after doctor, is how everyone remembers the sad stuff, the bad stuff, so vividly. Your brain presses record in HD. They can tell you the number of the room it happened in, on a labour ward they last saw a decade ago. The shoes the patient's husband was wearing, the song playing on the radio. Senior consultants' voices shake when they talk about their disasters – six-foot-tall former prop forwards on the verge of tears. A friend told me about a perimortem caesarean he performed: a mum dropped dead in front of him and he cut the baby out on the floor. It survived. 'You saved the wrong one! You saved the wrong one!' was all the dad could cry.

I'm not the right person to talk about dealing with grief though – that's not what this book is about. It's simply one doctor's experiences, some degree of insight on an individual level into what the job really entails.

But promise me this: next time the government takes its pickaxe to the NHS, don't just accept what the politicians try to feed you. Think about the toll the job takes on every healthcare professional, at home and at work. Remember they do an absolutely impossible job, to the very best of their abilities. Your time in hospital may well hurt them a lot more than it hurts you.

AN OPEN LETTER TO

THE SECRETARY OF STATE FOR HEALTH

Roger Fisher was a professor of law at Harvard University, who suggested back in 1981 that they should implant the American nuclear codes in the heart of a volunteer. If the President wanted to press the big red button and kill hundreds of thousands of innocent people, then first he'd have to take a butcher's knife and dig it out of the volunteer's chest himself; so that he realizes what death actually means first-hand, and understands the implications of his actions. Because the President would *never* press the button if he had to do that.

Similarly, you and your successor and their successors for ever more should have to work some shifts alongside junior doctors. Not the thing you already do, where a chief executive shows you round a brand-new ward that's gleaming like a space station. No: palliate a cancer patient; watch a trauma victim have their leg amputated; deliver a dead baby. Because I defy any human being, even you, to know what the job really entails and question a single doctor's motivation. If you knew, you would be applauding them, you'd be proud of them, you'd be humbled by them, and you'd be eternally grateful for everything they do.

The NHS isn't made up of hospitals, pharmacies and GP surgeries – it's made up of the people who work there. Be the politician in a generation who changes the stuck record and treats them with an ounce of respect.

Afterword

Presumably because I did something to mortally upset someone in the marketing department, upon publication of the hardback edition of *This is Going to Hurt*, I was despatched on a two-month-long UK book tour.

The tour had me pinballing around the country – from Crickhowell to St Boswells to Lytham St Annes – the only unifying factor being that I hadn't heard of any of them. Oh, and that none of them had any phone reception.

At the first hotel I stayed in, I asked for the Wifi code and the receptionist's finger waggled in the general direction of the communal computer in the hallway, with its Windows 95 operating system slowly drifting up the screen of a cathode-ray tube monitor, its vertical hold having died around the same time as Princess Diana. My room was agonizingly hot and someone in the floor above seemed to be constantly feeding ball-bearings through an industrial shredder. When the fire alarm went off at 2am, I wondered how badly burnt I'd have to be in order to get sent home from the tour.

And yet. These two months proved to be among the

most fun and fulfilling of my life. The book had clearly touched a nerve. Night after night I spoke in village halls packed with people who clearly cared passionately about the NHS – people who hadn't quite realized the extent of the pressures the staff who work there are under and the effect the job has on them. It was hugely humbling to be delivering this message, and even more encouraging that they listened.

I learned so much – that love for the health service runs deeper than any religion; that it transcends political belief and party membership; that if an audience has an average age over seventy then they probably won't enjoy the 'degloving' story.

At the end of every talk, I'd take questions, and the same one always came up: 'What can I do to help?' I spoke about the value of campaigning locally, of writing to papers, of contacting MPs, the power of social media, of joining progressive alliances and helping to crowd-fund legal challenges.

A few days into the tour, I started to notice just how many people would preface their questions and comments to me with 'my son/daughter/partner/neighbour/mother/best friend/uncle works for the NHS'. I began asking for a show of hands to see who had some kind of direct connection with NHS staff – there would only ever be one or two people in the room who kept their hands down. Often none. It makes sense, of course – the NHS employs the best part of 1.5 million people. And I realized there was a simpler, better answer to 'What can

I do to help?' One we can all do, that takes very little effort.

Ask them how their day was.

They'll say 'fine' and change the subject, or pull focus with some funny anecdote or other. But let them understand they've always got someone to talk to: someone who understands that the days are never actually just 'fine', that the nature of illness means more bad things happen at work than good. And keep on asking. Give them that opportunity to offload at the end of every shift, whether it's a tiny irritation, a rant or a full-on sob.

Chip away at the ingrained notion that doctors and nurses don't need to, or shouldn't, talk about these things – because that same ingrained notion is partly responsible for the huge rise in people leaving the profession, the rise in stress-related absence and illness among those who stay and the tragic rise in suicide amongst those who find it just too much. We all need someone to talk to. Don't let them bottle it up. Let them know you're there. Care for the carer.

Even though they've got a stethoscope round their neck and a decent line in gallows humour, they're still just that teenager who arbitrarily put a tick next to 'medicine' on their UCAS form. Just a human as fragile as anyone.

Extra Diary Entries

A lot of my diary entries didn't make it into the original edition of the book, and rightly so, it has to be said. Dozens just read 'Did caesarean number 357' or some such; many were impossible to justify legally because they'd clearly identify a patient, or in one instance described in precise detail the genitalia of a reality-show judge. Some we felt were topics that had been touched on enough elsewhere in the book and some were, in the words of my editor, 'tonally adrift', which I learned is publishing code for 'too disgusting'.

But apparently it's 'nice to include' some bonus material for the paperback edition, which I presume is publishing code for 'will hopefully sell some more copies'. You can decide for yourself into which category each of these rejected entries fell.

Tuesday, 17 May 2005

Patient CF has held the record for 'worst item inserted into penis' for three months, but now sadly his reign has come to an end. I was fairly confident that squirting a caulk gun down his urethra would have provided him with an unassailable lead – his story has certainly seen me through a lot of lulls in conversations. But, every bleep from A&E is a potential kingmaker, and we saw a new ruler crowned today.

Patient RD is a twenty-seven-year-old gentleman who attempted a new twist on an old classic to surprise his girlfriend on her birthday. He stripped naked, lay on his back on the kitchen table and smeared his body with chocolate sauce. He achieved an erection[*] then inserted and lit a thin green birthday candle. Unfortunately, his girlfriend didn't get a chance to see this ill-advised yet imaginative birthday tribute, as RD soon dissolved into the excruciating pain of hot wax dripping through his urethra and into his bladder. I presume as he blew out the candle he made a wish that the urology department would have a good plan as to how to remove the stick of wax melted deep into his cock.

Wednesday, 15 June 2005

Our ward has two computers for looking up results. In order to make it 'easier' to look them up while on a ward round, one of them has been replaced with a 'Computer on Wheels' aka 'CoW' aka 'laptop that's been welded to a barely modified Zimmer frame'. Quite

---

[*] This is a medical expression that has always surprised me; it's rather a small achievement in the grand scheme of things.

why they decided this leap in technology couldn't be in addition to the existing two computers I have no idea – but one of the PCs has been whisked away, and this has made life significantly worse.

There's an escalating war of early attendance to secure it, towels-on-deckchairs style, and today I'm in at 6:30 am to make sure the CoW is mine for the consultant round. Success! Only one slight downside – it's essentially unusable. The keyboard has metal keys, like an enormous cash machine keypad, making typing glacially slow. Plus it's got a comically short battery life, enough to see a couple of patients before it begins to flag and needs to be plugged in for an hour or two, rather negating its USP. I give it a week before it's scrapped, and a month before we find out that it cost the hospital sixteen billion pounds.

Friday, 20 July 2007

With Gordon Brown barely having unpacked his bags, it seems unfair to knock a point off a patient's Mental Test score for not knowing the name of the current Prime Minister. Although I feel like giving half a mark to the seventy-six-year-old lady who answered, 'You know, that Scottish wanker.'*

---

* I once put another of these standard dementia questions to a man in his nineties – 'Spell WORLD backwards.' He paused and said, 'As in "the planet" or "the past participle of 'to whirl'"?' Which was an excellent point.

Wednesday, 25 July 2007

Patient DM is eighty-three and complaining of vaginal pain and discharge. I try to gently pass a speculum. There's an ungodly smell, *plus ça change*. But what's that coming over the hill – is it a . . . ? Protruding is what can only really be a fetal leg bone. Good grief. I hurry away to vomit and speak to my senior registrar. He tells me to order a pelvic X-ray to work out exactly what and where these remains are, before we proceed.

Well, I was right about it being a leg. The X-ray confirmed quite a few legs in fact, plus a couple of wings. For once there's a merciful relief that it's just another tale of objects up vaginas – the thumping bassline of this job. She's clearly just got overexcited with a Bargain Bucket – perhaps there was free gravy? – and the contents are now decomposed. In a strange way, it's reassuring to know there's no upper limit on either age or revoltingness of object for this phenomenon.

Thursday, 20 May 2010

Not quite sure why patient BG has chosen to be referred to our department for menorrhagia* as she's spent a good five minutes explaining to me that she doesn't

---

* Menorrhagia means heavy periods, and no one has ever spelled it right first time. I literally typed it into Google and pasted in the correct spelling.

believe in modern medicine and there's nothing that can't be cured by homeopathy.*

I ask her how I can help today. Perhaps she wants me to witness her miraculous recovery first-hand as she necks her snake oil. 'I'm going to treat it with homeopathy. I just want a scan or something first – you know, to make sure it's nothing serious.'

Tuesday, 1 June 2010

It strikes me as common courtesy that if you're going to ask me to remove a Listerine cap from your vagina that got stuck during sex, you should warn me it's filled with your boyfriend's semen, not least so I can take measures to stop it splattering all over me upon removal, like high tide on the promenade.

Did it get stuck and you just thought, 'Fuck it, let's finish up and then I'll go to hospital'? Were you deliberately using it as a contraceptive device? Or did you just woefully misread the instructions on the Listerine bottle?

---

* I can sort of understand where other complementary 'therapies' are coming from, but homeopathy enthusiasts really baffle me. They're taking substances so dilute that every molecule of the 'medicine' is water. They clearly just want to believe. I guess it's an easier god to worship than some of the others, because you don't need to pray (until you're told it hasn't worked and you're actually dying), but to my mind, the only condition homeopathy can actually treat is thirst. Or being on fire, if applied topically.

Sunday, 11 July 2010

Watching an episode of *House* with H. This week, a woman whose asthma isn't improving is asked to demonstrate her inhaler technique; she proceeds to squirt it onto her neck like Joop. We laugh, though H suggests it's a little far-fetched. Not really: when I was a medical student on a GP placement, a man was attempting to manage his pet-hair-induced wheeze by puffing his inhaler onto the dog.

Friday, 23 July 2010

Life is one long fucking pub quiz and I am never on the right team. Two patients asked me questions today that I couldn't answer. First one was on labour ward triage – the patient's gums were bleeding. Diagnosis: gingivitis. Treatment: go to the dentist. She wondered why doctors learn about every single part of the body at medical school apart from the teeth, which are arbitrarily carved out of the syllabus and given to dentists. And why does it take the same length of time for them to study teeth as for us to study literally everything else? And why have teeth been singled out for non-doctors and not say, the ankle? The pancreas? Surely that would be no less weird? I bluffed my way through something colossally unconvincing about it being a historical peculiarity and pressed the test button on the side of my bleep to excuse myself.

I was consenting the second patient for caesarean section. When I asked if she had any questions, she said, 'What happens if there's a fire during my operation?' Perfectly reasonable but, worryingly, something no one from the hospital has ever trained us in. If only she'd asked me something that was covered in our hospital induction, like how to lift patients in a 'back safe' manner, or what colour bags used bed linen goes in.

We're at the end of a corridor on the third floor of an old building – I suspect the answer to her question involves either burning to death, or abseiling out of the window with an open abdomen. Or more likely, it's something the NHS would rather put its fingers in its ears about than actually address. Other such questions include, 'What would happen if all the doctors went home at the time they were contracted to?' and 'Why should anyone train to be a doctor any more?'

ACKNOWLEDGEMENTS

With love and thanks to Jess Cooper and Cath Summer-hayes at Curtis Brown. Jess, I'm sorry you had to read it so many times while heavily pregnant. To Francesca Main, my most incredible editor – I don't have the words. As usual.

To James, my co-pilot throughout.

To Drs Kay, Kay, Kay and Kay. Sophie – you'll be a much better obstetrician than I was. And Dan, you made the right choice by rebelling (and studying law). To my parents, Naomi and Stewart – love you really.

To everyone at Picador: particularly Ami Smithson, Paul Martinovic, Tom Noble, Paul Baggaley, Kish Widya-ratna, Christine Jones, Stuart Dwyer, Caitriona Row, Lucy Hine, Kate Tolley, Gillian Fitzgerald-Kelly, Rachel Mellor, Becky Fincham, and Anna Bond. And the indefatigable, inimitable Dusty Miller – the best publicist in the business.

To Mark Watson for making it all happen. To Jane Goldman for teaching me how to write long stuff. To Dan Swimer for the Knob-in-fan Persie joke. To Justin Myers for his wisdom of words. To Gerry Farrell for the title. To Stephen McCrum for that first TV writing job when I stumbled out of medicine. To Caroline Knight, my medical adviser ('Leave this bit out – it might actually stop people wanting children.'). To whoever makes Diplomático rum.

To so many former colleagues for jogging and sharing memories. Especially Drs Jones, Tanner, Gibson, Norbury, Trever, Henderson, van Hegan, Bonsall, Harvey, Heeps, Rehman, Bayliss, Saundershyphenvest, Laycock, McGinn, Lillie, Mansoori, Kupelian, Steingold, O'Neill, Biswas, Lieberman, Webster, Khan, Whitlock and Moore.

And to Anna Welander, Megan McCluskie, Karl Webster, Zoe Waterman, Nikki Williams, Tim Bittlestone, Mike Wozniak, Jackson Sargeant, Cath Gagon, James Seabright, Paul Sullivan, Annie Cullum, Michael Howard, Trish Farrell and everyone I've forgotten.

With no thanks whatsoever to Jeremy Hunt.

picador.com

blog
videos
interviews
extracts